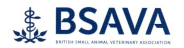

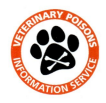

BSAVA/VPIS Guide to
Common Canine and Feline Poisons

Published by:
British Small Animal Veterinary Association,
Woodrow House, 1 Telford Way,
Waterwells Business Park, Quedgeley,
Gloucester GL2 2AB

A Company Limited by Guarantee in England
Registered Company No. 2837793
Registered as a Charity

ISBN 978-1-905319-45-9

Printed in India by Imprint Press
Printed on ECF paper made from sustainable forests   7935PUBS19

Other titles from BSAVA:

Manual of Avian Practice: A Foundation Manual
Manual of Canine & Feline Abdominal Imaging
Manual of Canine & Feline Abdominal Surgery
Manual of Canine & Feline Advanced Veterinary Nursing
Manual of Canine & Feline Anaesthesia and Analgesia
Manual of Canine & Feline Behavioural Medicine
Manual of Canine & Feline Cardiorespiratory Medicine
Manual of Canine & Feline Clinical Pathology
Manual of Canine & Feline Dentistry and Oral Surgery
Manual of Canine & Feline Dermatology
Manual of Canine & Feline Emergency and Critical Care
Manual of Canine & Feline Endocrinology
Manual of Canine & Feline Endoscopy and Endosurgery
Manual of Canine & Feline Fracture Repair and Management
Manual of Canine & Feline Gastroenterology
Manual of Canine & Feline Haematology and Transfusion Medicine
Manual of Canine & Feline Head, Neck and Thoracic Surgery
Manual of Canine & Feline Musculoskeletal Disorders
Manual of Canine & Feline Musculoskeletal Imaging
Manual of Canine & Feline Nephrology and Urology
Manual of Canine & Feline Neurology
Manual of Canine & Feline Oncology
Manual of Canine & Feline Ophthalmology
Manual of Canine & Feline Radiography and Radiology:
 A Foundation Manual
Manual of Canine & Feline Rehabilitation, Supportive and Palliative Care:
 Case Studies in Patient Management
Manual of Canine & Feline Reproduction and Neonatology
Manual of Canine & Feline Shelter Medicine: Principles of Health and
Welfare in a Multi-animal Environment
Manual of Canine & Feline Surgical Principles: A Foundation Manual
Manual of Canine & Feline Thoracic Imaging
Manual of Canine & Feline Ultrasonography
Manual of Canine & Feline Wound Management and Reconstruction
Manual of Canine Practice: A Foundation Manual
Manual of Exotic Pet and Wildlife Nursing
Manual of Exotic Pets: A Foundation Manual
Manual of Feline Practice: A Foundation Manual
Manual of Ornamental Fish
Manual of Practical Animal Care
Manual of Practical Veterinary Nursing
Manual of Psittacine Birds
Manual of Rabbit Medicine
Manual of Rabbit Surgery, Dentistry and Imaging
Manual of Raptors, Pigeons and Passerine Birds
Manual of Reptiles
Manual of Rodents and Ferrets
Manual of Small Animal Practice Management and Development
Manual of Wildlife Casualties

For further information on these and all BSAVA publications, please visit our
website: **www.bsava.com/shop**

Contents

Acknowledgements

The development of this book and the accompanying BSAVA/VPIS Poisons Triage Tool website has been a collaborative effort between the Veterinary Poisons Information Service (VPIS) and the British Small Animal Veterinary Association (BSAVA).

I would particularly like to thank my colleagues Karen Sturgeon, Leonard Hawkins and Nick Sutton for their written contributions, and especially Nicola Bates for her writing, editing and her project management of the content from the VPIS perspective.

Sophie Adamantos and Amanda Boag are to be thanked for their clinical expertise and for providing additional checking and editing, Lisa Archer for her marketing input and Elizabeth Dauncey for providing the plant photographs.

Finally I would like to acknowledge the efforts of the publishing team and IT development team at the BSAVA, with whom it has been a pleasure to work. Without them the whole venture would probably not have succeeded.

Alexander Campbell
Head of Service VPIS (1992–2012)

We are very grateful for the opportunity to update the text in this guide and ensure that it is accurate. This is the fourth time that we have revised the content and it is vital to continue doing so since our information and recommendations change as more information becomes available from our past cases and published literature. We would like to thank all the veterinary practices who support us through their memberships enabling us to continue this invaluable service, and to those practices who advise their clients to use our 24 hour triage service for owners, Animal PoisonLine. This relatively new public line ensures owners are armed with the right information in often very stressful situations. My thanks also go to my colleagues Nicola Bates and Tiffany Blackett for all their contributions and updates to this book.

Dr Nicola Robinson BSc MA VetMB MRCVS
Head of Service VPIS
April 2019

Foreword

The publication of this new guide marks the enormous advances that have been made into our understanding of poisoning in small animals. The development in knowledge owes a great deal to the inspirational work of Alex Campbell, former head of service, and the team at the Veterinary Poisons Information Service (VPIS), formed and supported initially by Guy's and St Thomas' NHS Foundation Trust, and now operating as a division of Emergency Scientific and Medical Services (ESMS). We also owe enormous thanks to thousands of veterinary surgeons who subscribe to the service and submit feedback forms to VPIS – without this feedback we would not have progressed to this point. The profession owes Alex a debt of gratitude for his extensive work in this field and his desire to improve the treatment of poisoned pets.

The *BSAVA/VPIS Guide to Common Canine and Feline Poisons* is designed to be a triage tool; the information contained has been compiled from the data sheets developed by VPIS over many years. The information will provide veterinary surgeons and nurses with a handy resource. We look forward to continuing our collaboration with VPIS in the future and supporting further work in this important area.

Andrew Ash BVetMed CertSAM MBA MRCVS
BSAVA President 2011–2012

(Foreword revised April 2019)

Introduction

This book contains brief summaries of information relating to poisoning of cats and dogs by commonly encountered substances. For each agent, information is given on toxicology, clinical effects, appropriate first aid and subsequent management and prognosis. This enables veterinary professionals to give appropriate guidance to clients that suspect their animals may have been poisoned. A traffic light system indicates the level of concern and urgency (see 'How to use this guide' page viii).

These summaries are **NOT** written with the aim of providing comprehensive advice about the management of any case. Many factors can influence how a case progresses and may affect management recommendations (dose, route(s) of exposure, time since exposure, duration of exposure, past medical history, breed or species susceptibility, environment, location, etc.).

For this reason these summaries should not be the sole information resource used to manage a poisoning case referred to a practice for treatment.

The inclusion of substances was determined by a review of enquiries made to VPIS and their case outcomes (where known).

- We have included substances of low or negligible toxicity about which VPIS receives many enquiries and for which presentation to a veterinary surgery is unlikely to be necessary.
- Other agents have been included owing to the number of exposures in the past and where the outcome has been variable.
- A few agents have also been included where exposures are relatively rare but toxicity is high and for which management may need to be speedy, complex or intensive, and where prognosis should be guarded. These latter categories are instances where reference to a veterinary poisons information service is strongly advised.

A bibliography of useful references, including case reports and case series, on the toxic effects of the substances summarized in this book is available on the VPIS website (**www.vpisglobal.com**).

A simple checklist is provided at the back of this book to guide veterinary staff of the type of information that is useful to gather about a possible poisoning case. The checklist can also be accessed online via the BSAVA/VPIS Poisons Triage Tool or the VPIS website. This can help ensure that the management advice provided will be specific to the individual case. This checklist can be used to help complete case follow-up questionnaires or the case submission form.

VPIS exists to provide specific advice, compliant with UK veterinary medicine legislation, for each and every case referred to it on its own individual merits. The information given in this book has been compiled by VPIS in line with these considerations.

Every effort has been made to ensure that the information within these summaries is both accurate and current. Please be aware that online information may be updated or changed in the light of any relevant publications, VPIS cases and systematic revisions. BSAVA Members have access to the online BSAVA/VPIS Poisons Triage Tool via **www.bsava.com** and are recommended to check this for updated or additional information. For information about joining BSAVA, please visit the Membership page at **www.bsava.com**.

The VPIS is always keen to receive feedback on poisoning cases even if not consulted, to build on its extensive internal database of past referrals. Of particular interest are complex, serious and unusual cases, or where toxicity information was limited. Even if the animal remained asymptomatic this information is still useful. To submit information on a poisoning case to VPIS, please visit **www.vpisglobal.com**. VPIS follows up some cases using a postal questionnaire, in an attempt to determine treatments given, clinical course and outcome.

This resource is the result of an exciting collaborative venture between BSAVA and VPIS. We hope that it will provide a valuable resource and we welcome your comments and suggestions.

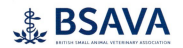

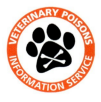

How to use this guide

The poisons monographs are divided into canine (blue-headed pages) and feline (mauve-headed pages). Please note that data in entries for one animal species will not always be applicable to another species – some animals respond to different poisons in very different ways.

Within each section the monographs are listed alphabetically. Please note that generic names are used for all pharmaceutical agents; trade and proprietary names are not included. Plants and animals are listed under both common and Latin names. Please use the Index to find poisons listed by their alternative names.

Each poison monograph follows the same essential format.

Alternative names

- This notes alternative names, such as common names for plants; for example, daffodil is the common name for *Narcissus* species.
- Where an entry refers to a group of agents (e.g. anticoagulant rodenticides) a list is given of the various compounds for which the subsequent guidance would be appropriate.
- Please note that trade, brand and proprietary names are not used. To determine the contents of a particular product you should refer to the packaging or contact VPIS. VPIS has many resources available to determine the contents of commercial products.
- Alternative names are included in the Index.

Description/Source

- This provides a description of the agent and how it might be presented. Where medicines, pesticides and household chemicals are involved, information is provided on the intended uses of the agents, indications of how they might be presented or packaged, and in what likely concentrations.
- For plants there will be a brief description of the appearance of the plant parts and how they may vary with season, plus notes on individual species where appropriate.

Toxicology

This section describes how and why the agent is thought to be toxic (if this is known). It may give some indications or measures of toxicity.

Risk factors

- Some breeds are known to be more affected than others by certain poisons.

- In some cases previous exposures to the specific or similar agents may increase the risk.
- Pre-existing disease states (e.g. renal insufficiency) can also impact on responses to certain substances. If the animal exposed fits into any of these categories, then immediate discussion with VPIS is advised.

Clinical effects

- **Onset:** a rough guide as to the likely time it would take for clinical signs to appear. This can be useful in determining how urgent referral to a surgery should be, or whether an otherwise asymptomatic animal need attend at all.
- **Common signs:** a listing of the clinical signs most commonly reported, described or characteristic of the particular intoxication. These are usually listed in a general order of increased severity, although this may depend on dose.
- **Other signs:** less frequently observed signs or those that occur in only the most severe cases.

Treatment

The advice in this section is NOT intended to be comprehensive guidance to the management of any case, as that will depend on many factors. It should not be the sole information resource used to manage a poisoning case referred to a practice for treatment. Contact details for VPIS are given on the inside front cover.

- This section indicates when decontamination is appropriate. Details of methods are available in the Decontamination section at the back of the book.
- General information is given on treatment modalities that may subsequently be necessary.
- Where specific antidotal therapies may be required, dosing information is provided.

Prognosis

- This provides indication(s) of the likely prognosis of a poisoning case involving the agent in question. This may vary according to dose, case history and even speed of presentation and level of veterinary intervention.
- *In instances where prognosis is guarded or poor, every effort should be made to intervene to ensure the most favourable case outcome is achieved.*
- *Never give up unless you have to!*
- *VPIS is always there to guide you through the management of animals with poisoning. On-call veterinary emergency and critical care consultants are also available, if required.*

Alert status

As a handy visual reference for those cases where a very quick response may be needed, we have applied a 'traffic light' system for classifying the risks of each agent/types of agent.

Red

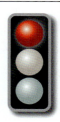

- Exposure to the agent in question in the particular species may result in severe or life-threatening clinical signs and prognosis may be guarded. However, prompt and aggressive treatment could (depending on the agent) change this. Some toxicities can be treated but others are difficult to treat successfully.
- The animal should be taken to a veterinary surgery as a matter of urgency, with any other evidential material (product packaging, etc.).
- VPIS should be consulted about the case as soon as is practicable.

Amber

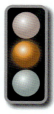

- Exposures to the agent are relatively common, and although most cases have a favourable outcome some fatal cases have occurred.
- The animal should ideally be taken to a veterinary surgery as soon as possible for full veterinary review.
- VPIS can give advice as to the likelihood of severe poisoning.

Green

- Exposures to the agent are common.
- The substance is considered by VPIS to be of low or negligible toxicity.
- No obvious signs of illness may occur; where they do occur, they are likely to be mild and transient.
- The animal is unlikely to need to attend a veterinary surgery unless there are extenuating circumstances or unusual signs have occurred.
- The general management advice given in 'Treatment' should be followed.

ACE inhibitor exposure in dogs

A
B
C
D
E
F
G
H
I
J
K
L
M
N
O
P
Q
R
S
T
U
V
W
X
Y
Z

Alternative names

Examples: benazepril, captopril, cilazapril, enalapril, fosinopril, imidapril, lisinopril, moexipril, perindopril, quinapril, ramipril

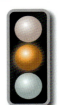

Description/Source

Used in the treatment of heart failure, hypertension, diabetic nephropathy and in the prophylaxis of cardiovascular events in humans. In dogs they are used for congestive heart failure, hypertension and protein-losing nephropathy; used in cats with chronic renal failure.

Toxicology

Angiotensin converting enzyme (ACE) catalyses the conversion of angiotensin I to angiotensin II. ACE inhibitors block the action of ACE, resulting in a decrease of angiotensin II and leading to vasodilation, lowered blood pressure and increased cardiac output. Most of these drugs are well tolerated in dogs and cases of severe toxicity are rare.

Risk factors

None known.

Clinical effects

Onset

Within 6 hours.

Common signs

Vomiting, diarrhoea, hypotension and tachycardia.

Other signs

Renal failure.

Treatment

- Empty the stomach and give activated charcoal (see Decontamination).
- Symptomatic and supportive care.
- Ensure adequate hydration.

Prognosis

Excellent.

Adder bite in dogs

Description/Source

The European adder (*Vipera berus*) is the only venomous snake native to the UK. The adult is about 50 cm long, pale grey/green to dark brown with characteristic black/brown dorsal zig-zag patterning (not obvious if very dark). Its preferred habitat is heaths, sand dunes, moorlands and woodland margins. It is a protected species. Adders usually bite only when provoked. Bites are more frequent during the summer.

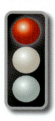

Toxicology

Adder venom is a complex mixture of proteins that causes the release of pharmacologically active substances such as histamine, serotonin, bradykinin and prostaglandins. It also has direct effects on heart and blood vessels and on the release of cytolytic and haemolytic factors.

Risk factors

None known.

Clinical effects

Onset

Rapid, usually within 2 hours.

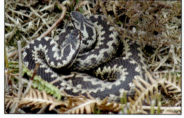

Vipera berus.
Courtesy of Matthew Rendle

Common signs

Puncture wounds may be visible.
Localized painful swelling may spread and become haemorrhagic. Bites to the muzzle can affect the dog's ability to eat, drink and thermoregulate. Also mental status changes, varying from lethargy and depression to coma, tachycardia, hyperthermia, lameness, bruising, pale mucous membranes, hypersalivation, vomiting, and panting.

Other signs

Shock, collapse, renal, hepatic and cardiac effects and coagulopathy.

Treatment

- Speed is essential.
- Keep the dog still and quiet if possible.
- **Leave the bite site alone.** Immobilize affected limb. **Use of incisions, suction and tourniquets is not recommended.**
- Consider specific antivenom at the earliest opportunity, and definitely in all cases where bites are on the muzzle or facial region.

- Symptomatic and supportive care.
- Steroids should not be used and antibiotics should only be given if there is evidence of infection.
- In case of haemorrhage, check for possible coagulopathy.

Prognosis

Favourable in mild to moderate cases. Guarded if severe signs occur.

Aesculus hippocastanum exposure in dogs

Alternative names

Horse chestnut, conker

Description/Source

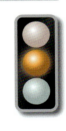

A deciduous tree growing to about 25 metres, common in parks and urban areas. Fruits are large spiny, green, yellow or brown capsules containing one or more shiny brown seeds (conkers), which ripen from August to October.

Toxicology

All parts of the plant contain aesculin, a saponin glycoside. The bark, leaves and flowers are the most toxic. The seed contains starch and approximately 5% aesculin.

Risk factors

None known.

Clinical effects

Onset

Usually within 6 hours.

Common signs

Vomiting, diarrhoea, hypersalivation, abdominal tenderness, polydipsia, anorexia and dehydration.

Other signs

Obstruction of the gastrointestinal tract can occur.

Conkers (from *Aesculus hippocastanum*).
©Elizabeth Dauncey

Treatment

- Gut decontamination is generally not required, as vomiting often occurs spontaneously.

A B C D E F G H I J K L M N O P Q R S T U V W X Y Z

- Ensure adequate hydration and give anti-emetics if required.
- Symptomatic and supportive care.

Prognosis

Favourable.

Allium species exposure in dogs

Description/Source

A large group of mostly perennial bulbous herbs: *Allium ampeloprasum* (leek); *Allium cepa* (onion, shallot); *Allium fistulosum* (spring onion); *Allium moly* (golden garlic, lily leek); *Allium sativum* (garlic); *Allium schoenoprasum* (chive); *Allium ursinum* (wild garlic, wood garlic, ramsons); *Allium vineale* (field garlic, wild garlic, crow garlic); ornamental allium. They have a characteristic strong aroma when bruised or crushed. The leaves and bulbs of many species are used in cooking (fresh, dried and powdered); some are also grown for their ornamental flowers.

Toxicology

Allium species contain a variety of organosulphoxides. Trauma to the plants converts these to a variety of organic sulphur compounds that deplete glucose-6-phosphate dehydrogenase (G6PD) within erythrocytes, resulting in Heinz body formation and anaemia.

Risk factors

Japanese and Korean breeds.

Clinical effects

Onset

Sometimes within 24 hours but more commonly after several days.

Common signs

Gastrointestinal effects (inappetence, vomiting, abdominal discomfort and diarrhoea) and Heinz body anaemia.

Other signs

Methaemoglobinaemia and jaundice.

Treatment

- Empty the stomach and give activated charcoal (see Decontamination).

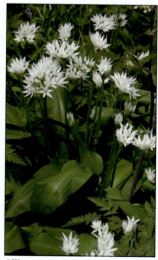

Allium sp.
©Elizabeth Dauncey

- Monitor haematological parameters.
- Ensure adequate hydration.
- Symptomatic and supportive care.

Prognosis

Favourable.

Allopurinol exposure in dogs

Description/Source

A xanthine oxidase inhibitor used in the prophylactic management of recurrent uric acid uroliths and hyperuricosuric calcium oxalate urolithiasis. In humans it is used in the prophylactic management of idiopathic gout and prevention of calcium oxalate and uric acid renal stones.

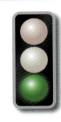

Toxicology

Allopurinol decreases the formation of uric acid by inhibiting xanthine oxidase, which catalyses the conversion of hypoxanthine to xanthine and of xanthine to uric acid. It is well tolerated in overdose.

Risk factors

None known.

Clinical effects

Onset

Probably within a few hours.

Common signs

Vomiting, diarrhoea and abdominal tenderness.

Other signs

Excitability and polydipsia may occur.

Treatment

- Gut decontamination is not required unless ingestion is substantial (see Decontamination).
- Ensure adequate hydration and give anti-emetics if required.
- Symptomatic and supportive care.

Prognosis

Excellent.

A B C D E F G H I J K L M N O P Q R S T U V W X Y Z

Alphachloralose exposure in dogs

For exposure in cats – see page 120

Alternative name

Chloralose

Description/Source

A rodenticide for mice and rats; also used to control pest birds. Baits are available in various forms including wheat or bran granules containing 2 to 4%. Professional products may be more concentrated.

Toxicology

Alphachloralose possesses both stimulant and depressant properties. At low exposures it causes excitation by suppressing the descending inhibitory mechanisms in the nervous system. At higher doses it acts as a central nervous system depressant through neuronal suppression in the ascending reticular activating system.

Risk factors

None known.

Clinical effects

Onset

Usually within 1 to 2 hours.

Common signs

Initially hyperactivity and ataxia. Then hypersalivation, drowsiness, weakness, hyperaesthesia, hypothermia, shallow respiration, coma and convulsions.

Other signs

Respiratory failure and hyperthermia (from repeated convulsions).

Treatment

- Empty the stomach (see Decontamination).
- Activated charcoal is not useful.
- Monitor respiration and temperature.
- Diazepam can be used for tremors, twitching or convulsions but other drugs may be required (e.g. pentobarbital, phenobarbital).
- Warming measures if patient is hypothermic and cooling measures if patient is hyperthermic.
- Symptomatic and supportive care.

Prognosis

Favourable with prompt treatment.

Amitraz exposure in dogs

Description/Source

A topical formamidine ectoparasiticide used for lice, fleas and ticks on dogs.

Toxicology

The mechanism of action of amitraz is not known, but appears to be similar to that of alpha-2 adrenergic agonists (e.g. xylazine, clonidine). Toxicity occurs after topical overdose or ingestion. Cardiovascular effects are due to activation of alpha-2 adrenergic receptors. Hyperglycaemia (and resultant polyuria) is due to inhibition of insulin release.

Risk factors

Chihuahua (risk of idiosyncratic reactions).

Clinical effects

Onset

1 to 2 hours.

Common signs

Depression, vomiting, pale mucous membranes, inappetence, diarrhoea, ataxia, shaking, dyspnoea, bradycardia, hypotension, hypothermia, dilated pupils and collapse.

Other signs

Hypertension, hyperglycaemia and subsequent polyuria.

Treatment

- **Emesis is best avoided; α_2-adrenergic agonists (e.g. xylazine, medetomidine or dexmedetomidine) should not be given.**
- Give activated charcoal (see Decontamination).
- If appropriate, decontaminate the skin by washing with a mild detergent and lukewarm water (see Decontamination).
- Monitor blood pressure, temperature, heart rate and blood glucose.
- Atipamezole can be used to reverse sedation and bradycardia.
- Symptomatic and supportive care.

Prognosis

Favourable.

Amoxicillin exposure in dogs

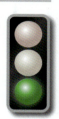

Alternative name

Amoxycillin

Description/Source

Broad-spectrum penicillin antibiotic, often combined with clavulanic acid (amoxicillin/clavulanate).

Toxicology

Amoxicillin is of low acute toxicity. Gastrointestinal signs can occur at therapeutic doses but are more likely with overdose.

Risk factors

Renal impairment; hypersensitivity to penicillins.

Clinical effects

Onset

Gastrointestinal signs within a few hours of ingestion; renal effects can also occur rapidly in some cases.

Common signs

Vomiting, anorexia, diarrhoea and abdominal discomfort. Hypersensitivity reactions with maculopapular or urticarial rash and pyrexia can occur but are rare in animals.

Other signs

Renal failure, haematuria and crystalluria can occur but are rare.

Treatment

- Gut decontamination is not required.
- Ensure adequate hydration.
- Monitor renal function if required.
- Hypersensitivity reactions should be managed conventionally.
- Symptomatic and supportive care.

Prognosis

Excellent.

Anticoagulant rodenticide exposure in dogs

Alternative names

Examples: brodifacoum, bromadiolone, chlorophacinone, coumatetralyl, difenacoum, difethialone, diphacinone, flocoumafen, warfarin

Description/Source

These compounds are used in many rodenticide preparations. Amateur products are usually of low concentration (commonly 0.0025% w/w) but professional products may be more concentrated. Warfarin has medicinal use in management of human thromboembolic disorders.

Toxicology

Competitively inhibits hepatic vitamin K1 epoxide reductase. Clotting factors II, VII, IX and X become depleted and hepatic prothrombin synthesis is impaired.

Risk factors

Other coagulopathies; hypothyroidism; pre-existing hepatic disease; previous exposure to these compounds.

Clinical effects

Onset

Usually within 3–5 (sometimes 7) days. Prothrombin time (PT) is prolonged after at least 36 hours.

Common signs

Non-specific signs with lethargy, weakness, anorexia, cough, depression and pale mucous membranes. Internal bleeding, particularly into the lungs, is more common than external bleeding.

Other signs

Depends on the location of the haemorrhage. Risk of hypovolaemic shock.

Treatment

- Empty the stomach and give activated charcoal (see Decontamination).
- In asymptomatic dogs
  - **Either** give vitamin K1 for at least 21 days and assess the PT 48 hours after the last dose **or** assess clotting 48–72 hours after ingestion and then give vitamin K1 for at least 21 days if the PT is prolonged.
  - If there is concern that exposure may be chronic either start vitamin K1 immediately or check the PT immediately and then 24–48 hours later.

- In symptomatic dogs start vitamin K1 immediately and admit for at least 24 hours.
- In severe cases transfusions of plasma or whole blood will be required.

Prognosis

Favourable in animals with mild clinical signs controlled with vitamin K1. Poor in dogs with severe, uncontrolled haemorrhage.

Antihistamine exposure in dogs

Alternative names

Examples: acrivastine, cetirizine, chlorphenamine, cinnarizine, clemastine, cyclizine, cyproheptadine, desloratadine, diphenhydramine, fexofenadine, hydroxyzine, levocetirizine, loratadine, meclozine, mizolastine, pizotifen

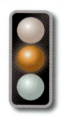

Description/Source

Widely used in human and veterinary medicine for allergic disorders and motion sickness.

Toxicology

Antihistamines act as reversible, competitive inhibitors of the interaction of histamine with H1 receptors. The first generation (sedating) antihistamines are lipophilic, have cholinergic effects and cross the blood–brain barrier, causing sedation. The second generation (non-sedating) antihistamines are lipophobic and tend to cause less central nervous system and cholinergic effects at therapeutic doses; they exhibit fewer effects on H2 receptors and therefore have reduced anticholinergic and antiserotinergic adverse effects.

Risk factors

None known.

Clinical effects

Onset

4 to 7 hours.

Common signs

Vomiting, hypersalivation, incoordination, ataxia, lethargy, tremor, depression, hyperthermia, tachycardia and weakness. In severe cases coma, convulsions, hypotension and respiratory depression may occur.

Other signs
Some animals may exhibit hyperactivity and hyperaesthesia.

Treatment
- Empty the stomach and give activated charcoal (see Decontamination).
- Symptomatic and supportive care.
- Ensure adequate hydration.

Prognosis
Favourable.

Arachis hypogaea exposure in dogs

Alternative names
Peanuts, groundnuts, monkey nuts, earthnuts, jack nuts

Description/Source
A legume native to South and Central America. Commonly available as a food and in peanut butter, peanut oil and sweets. Peanuts are also available salted (see Sodium chloride) or chocolate-coated (see Chocolate).

Toxicology
Most dogs that ingest peanuts develop only gastrointestinal signs. Occasionally dogs develop neurotoxicity but the cause of this, and other effects, is unknown. There are no cases of peanut poisoning in dogs reported in the literature. It is possible that convulsions result from the ingestion of the salt on salted peanuts. Peanuts are also a potential source of aflatoxins but this is characterized by liver damage, not neurotoxicity.

Risk factors
None known.

Clinical effects

Onset
Within a few hours.

Common signs
Most dogs develop gastrointestinal signs with vomiting, diarrhoea and abdominal discomfort.

Other signs

Convulsions, tremor and restlessness have been reported (but this may be due to salt on salted peanuts).

Treatment

- Consider emptying the stomach if a large quantity has been ingested (see Decontamination).
- Sedation may be required.
- Symptomatic and supportive care.

Prognosis

Favourable.

Aspirin overdose in dogs

Alternative name

Acetylsalicylic acid

Description/Source

An anti-inflammatory, antipyretic analgesic also used as an anti-platelet drug. Aspirin is often found in combination with other analgesics including paracetamol and caffeine. Other salicylates, such as methyl salicylate (oil of wintergreen), are used as topical anti-inflammatory analgesics.

Toxicology

In **overdose** salicylate stimulates the respiratory centre, causing hyperventilation and a respiratory alkalosis. The body compensates by excreting bicarbonate, sodium and potassium ions and water in urine, resulting in electrolyte imbalance, dehydration and a decrease in the buffering capacity of the body. This allows the development of an anion gap metabolic acidosis, which enhances transfer of the salicylate ion across the blood-brain barrier, resulting in central nervous system effects. Salicylate uncouples oxidative phosphorylation, decreasing adenine triphosphate (ATP) production. There is increased oxygen utilization and increased production of carbon dioxide (contributing to hyperventilation) and lactate (contributing to metabolic acidosis). The energy that should be used to produce ATP is dissipated as heat.

Risk factors

None known.

Clinical effects

Onset

Gastrointestinal effects often occur within 2 hours.

Common signs

Depression, vomiting, anorexia, hyperthermia, tachypnoea, respiratory alkalosis then metabolic acidosis. Haematemesis, gastric ulceration and gastrointestinal bleeding may occur but are more common with chronic administration.

Other signs

Hypernatraemia, hypokalaemia, pulmonary and cerebral oedema, coma, convulsions and renal damage.

Treatment

- Empty the stomach and give activated charcoal (see Decontamination).
- Ensure adequate hydration and give anti-emetics if required.
- Monitor urea and electrolytes if required.
- Monitor blood gases if acid–base derangements are suspected.
- Gastric protectants are recommended (see BSAVA Formulary).
- Symptomatic and supportive care.

Prognosis

Favourable with supportive care.

Baclofen exposure in dogs

Description/Source

Baclofen is a skeletal muscle relaxant used in human medicine for chronic muscle spasm or control of muscle spasticity (e.g. in multiple sclerosis, spinal cord injuries, cerebral palsy).

Toxicology

Baclofen inhibits the central nervous system reflexes, with effects often being more pronounced in the spinal cord. It binds to presynaptic gamma-aminobutyric acid-B (GABA-B) receptors, reducing transmitter release, possibly through a reduction in presynaptic calcium ion influx. It may also have a post-synaptic effect mediated through an increase in potassium ion permeability, which changes regulation of neuronal excitability.

Risk factors

None known.

Clinical effects

Onset

Rapid, usually within 1 hour of ingestion.

Common signs

Excitability, hypersalivation, constricted pupils, vocalization, weakness, ataxia, twitching, tremor, bradycardia, pale mucous membranes, drowsiness, loss of swallowing reflexes and collapse.

Other signs

Cyanosis, coma, convulsions, shock, hypothermia, tachycardia and respiratory distress/hypoventilation.

Treatment

- Empty the stomach and give activated charcoal (see Decontamination).
- Diazepam or acepromazine may be needed for muscle tremors or to control convulsions.
- Artificial ventilation may be required.
- Consider use of intravenous lipid emulsion in a severe case unresponsive to other therapies.
- Symptomatic and supportive care.

Prognosis

Guarded.

Barbiturate exposure in dogs

Alternative names

Examples: pentobarbital, phenobarbital, primidone

Description/Source

Barbiturates are used as anticonvulsants, sedatives and anaesthetics. Pentobarbital is also used for euthanasia.

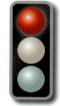

Toxicology

Barbiturates reversibly depress the activity of all excitable tissue. They also affect the peripheral nervous system, depressing transmission in autonomic ganglia and reducing nicotinic excitation by choline esters. Sedative doses of barbiturates have little effect on the cardiovascular system but in overdose they cause direct depression of cardiac contractility. In the gastrointestinal tract barbiturates decrease tonus of the musculature and the amplitude of the rhythmic contractions, causing reduced gut motility.

Risk factors

None known.

Clinical effects

Onset

Usually 1 to 8 hours, often 4 to 6 hours.

Common signs

Central nervous system depression with drowsiness, ataxia, disorientation, hypothermia and, in severe cases, coma, respiratory depression, hypotension and cardiovascular collapse. There is also decreased gut motility and ileus.

Other signs

Renal failure, anaemia, leucopenia, thrombocytopenia and a transient decrease in PCV and haemoglobin.

Treatment

- Empty the stomach and give activated charcoal (see Decontamination).
- Monitor respiratory rate and blood pressure if possible.
- The usual care of a comatose animal should be employed, with monitoring of vital signs and regular turning.
- Warming measures may be required.
- In animals with significant central nervous system depression, monitor the full blood count and liver function.
- Doxapram can be used to stimulate the respiratory and cardiac systems but the effect may be temporary.
- In animals with respiratory depression oxygen may be given with ventilation if required.
- Intravenous fluids can be used for hypotension.
- Symptomatic and supportive care.

Prognosis

Favourable with supportive care.

Battery exposure in dogs

Description/Source

Power supplies for calculators, electronic games, watches, hearing aids, photographic equipment, remote controls, mobile phones and pagers, etc. There are five principal chemical types: mercury; lithium; alkaline-manganese; silver; and zinc-air. Most batteries contain alkaline hydroxide solutions, regardless of their chemical type.

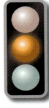

Toxicology

Batteries may cause: electrical burns; chemical burns as a result of current-induced alkali production or leakage of alkali content; or chemical toxicity as a result of absorption of leaked contents. Some small button/disc batteries used to contain mercuric chloride but these are now banned in many countries. Severe effects are rare; most undamaged batteries that are ingested pass through the gut intact.

Risk factors

None known.

Clinical effects

Onset

Variable, depending on whether the battery is chewed or swallowed whole.

Common signs

Hypersalivation and vomiting.

Other signs

Oral or tongue inflammation, ulceration and burns, abdominal discomfort and melaena. Risk of perforation if lodged in the gastrointestinal tract.

Treatment

- Determine type of battery.
- **Do not induce vomiting.**
- Asymptomatic animals can probably be observed at home.
- If signs suggestive of irritation occur gastroprotectants and analgesia can be given.
- If the battery may have lodged or there are significant gastrointestinal signs, then X-rays should be taken to determine the location and condition of the battery.
- If the battery is lodged in the stomach or beyond and clinical signs are significant it should be removed via endoscopy or surgery.
- If the battery is lodged in the oesophagus it should be removed immediately.

Prognosis

Favourable.

Bendroflumethiazide exposure in dogs

Alternative name

Bendrofluazide

Description/Source

A thiazide diuretic used in human medicine for oedema and hypertension.

Toxicology

Bendroflumethiazide exerts its diuretic effect by inhibition of sodium reabsorption from the distal convoluted tubule.

Risk factors

None known. Possibly volume depletion, hypotension or renal impairment.

Clinical effects

Onset

Limited information in animals but in humans diuresis occurs within 1 to 2 hours.

Common signs

Most animals remain asymptomatic, but polyuria, polydipsia and drowsiness may occur.

Other signs

Excessive fluid loss may lead to dehydration and electrolyte imbalance.

Treatment

- Empty the stomach and give activated charcoal (see Decontamination).
- Ensure adequate hydration.
- Monitor renal function.
- Symptomatic and supportive care.

Prognosis

Favourable.

Benzodiazepine exposure in dogs

For exposure in cats – see page 122

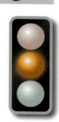

Alternative name

Examples: alprazolam, bromazepam, chlordiazepoxide, clobazam, clonazepam, clorazepate, diazepam, flunitrazepam, flurazepam, loprazolam, lorazepam, lormetazepam, midazolam, nitrazepam, oxazepam, temazepam

Description/Source

Benzodiazepines are used as sedatives, anxiolytics, anticonvulsants and premedicants.

Toxicology

Benzodiazepines enhance the effect of the inhibitory neurotransmitter gamma-aminobutyric acid (GABA).

Risk factors

None known.

Clinical effects

Onset

Usually within 2 hours.

Common signs

Ataxia, incoordination and drowsiness.

Other signs

Tremor, lethargy, depression, weakness, vomiting, hypothermia, nystagmus, disorientation, polydipsia and polyphagia, coma, hypotension and respiratory depression. Some animals develop paradoxical stimulation, with hyperactivity, hyperaesthesia, agitation, restlessness, aggression and hyperthermia.

Treatment

- Give activated charcoal (see Decontamination).
- Symptomatic and supportive care.
- Flumazenil could be considered in animals with severe respiratory or central nervous system depression. *Dosage*: 0.01–0.02 mg/kg i.v., repeated after about 30 minutes, if required.

Prognosis

Favourable.

Beta-blocker exposure in dogs

Alternative names

Examples: acebutolol, atenolol, bisoprolol, carvedilol, celiprolol, esmolol, labetalol, metoprolol, nadolol, nebivolol, oxprenolol, pindolol, propranolol, sotalol, timolol

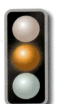

Description/Source

Used in dogs for tachycardia and as an anti-arrhythmic. In humans they are used for hypertension, angina, myocardial infarction, arrhythmias, heart failure, anxiety and prophylaxis of migraine.

Toxicology

Beta-blockers exert negative inotropic and chronotropic effects at the beta-1 adrenoceptors. They increase constriction of bronchi and dilatation of blood vessels and decrease the breakdown of glycogen. Variations in cardioselectivity, partial agonist activity, membrane stabilizing activity and lipophilicity influence the clinical effects. In **overdose**, lowered blood pressure and heart rate are more pronounced and therefore hazardous.

Risk factors

Pre-existing heart disease.

Clinical effects

Onset

Within 6 hours for standard release preparations. Within 12 hours for sustained release preparations.

Common signs

Hypotension and bradycardia (tachycardia, if beta-blocker with partial agonist activity ingested e.g. pindolol), drowsiness, respiratory depression, convulsions and hypoglycaemia.

Other signs

Hyperkalaemia, pulmonary oedema and arrhythmias.

Treatment

- Empty the stomach and give activated charcoal (see Decontamination). Give repeat doses of activated charcoal if a sustained release preparation has been ingested.
- Symptomatic and supportive care.
- Hypotension should initially be treated with intravenous fluids. Take care in patients with heart disease. Hypotension associated with bradycardia may respond to atropine.

- If these fail then consider high dose insulin/dextrose therapy and/or intravenous lipid emulsion.

Prognosis

Favourable with treatment.

Blue-green algae exposure in dogs

Alternative name

Cyanobacteria

Description/Source

Primitive organisms with characteristics of both bacteria and algae. They are capable of photosynthesis, the chlorophyll giving them the observed blue-green colour in many cases, and some are also able to fix gaseous nitrogen. They are found in fresh, brackish and marine water bodies throughout the UK. In any location there may be many different types co-existing. Under favourable conditions (sunny weather, high water temperature and abundant nutrients, especially nitrogen and phosphorus) the blue-green algae may form massive growths or 'blooms'. Blooms occur most commonly in late spring, summer and early autumn.

Toxicology

There are many species of blue-green algae; only some produce toxic compounds. These toxins have a high acute toxicity, and exposure frequently results in fatality. Death is usually very rapid. It is calculated that concentrated scums at the edges of water bodies present a toxic or lethal dose of blue-green algal toxins in a very small fluid volume. The mechanism of toxicity depends on the species: some contain or produce hepatotoxins, others neurotoxins. Clinical effects are wide ranging as they depend on the type(s) of toxins involved; exposure may involve several different species of blue-green alga simultaneously. Most animals with suspected exposure remain asymptomatic, but this may be either because they have not actually been exposed or because the algae observed are not toxic.

Risk factors

None known.

Clinical effects

Onset
Within 1 hour (neurotoxic) or within 24 hours (hepatotoxic).

Common signs
Variable, depending on species/toxins. Gastrointestinal upset (vomiting, haematemesis, abdominal tenderness), dermatitis, neurotoxic (tremors, bradycardia, tachypnoea, twitching, muscle rigidity, ataxia, paralysis, respiratory distress, convulsions and coma) and/or hepatotoxic effects (weakness, haemorrhage, hypotension, elevated liver enzymes and jaundice).

Other signs
Hepatotoxins may cause nephritis and liver failure.

Treatment
- Empty the stomach and give activated charcoal (see Decontamination).
- If appropriate, decontaminate the skin by washing with a mild detergent and lukewarm water (see Decontamination).
- Ensure adequate hydration.
- Monitor hepatic and renal function.
- Give liver protectants (S-adenosylmethionine, acetylcysteine).
- Administer anticonvulsants if required.
- Administer atropine if bradycardic.
- Symptomatic and supportive care.

Prognosis
Poor in symptomatic cases.

Borax exposure in dogs

Alternative names
Sodium borate, sodium tetraborate, disodium tetraborate

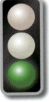

Description/Source
Found in many ant or cockroach killer preparations (usually sugary solutions containing 5–7% borax). Borates have limited use in mouthwashes, contact lens solutions, liquid medical preparations such as eye drops, and some soaps and detergents.

Toxicology

The mechanism of toxicity is unknown; borates prevent epithelialization and are generally considered to be cytotoxic to all cells. Concentrated borax solutions are irritant to skin and mucous membranes. Severe poisoning from ingestion of a domestic pesticide is unlikely.

Risk factors

None known.

Clinical effects

Onset

Usually within 2 hours.

Common signs

Buccal and gastrointestinal irritation, particularly vomiting, diarrhoea, abdominal tenderness and salivation.

Other signs

Shivering, shaking, tremors, ataxia, drowsiness and depression have been reported. Rarely pyrexia, polydipsia, convulsions and collapse. Skin exposures may result in erythema.

Treatment

- Gut decontamination is probably not necessary following ingestion of borax at concentrations up to 10% in strength.
- Symptomatic and supportive care.

Prognosis

Favourable.

Buprenorphine exposure in dogs

Description/Source

Buprenorphine is a derivative of the morphine alkaloid thebaine. It is an opioid analgesic that is used to relieve moderate to severe pain in both humans and animals. In humans it is also used in the treatment of opioid dependence. Common preparations include sublingual tablets, transdermal patches and injectable forms. The injectable form is authorized for use in dogs and cats. Parenteral buprenorphine has twice the duration of action of morphine and is about 30 times more potent.

Toxicology

Buprenorphine is a partial agonist opioid, acting at the mu opioid receptor that mediates its analgesic effect. It also has antagonistic activity at the kappa opioid receptor. The kappa opioid receptor is complex but is involved in perception of pain. Buprenorphine has a relatively long duration of action and effects from the drug may persist for several hours or even days.

Risk factors

None known.

Clinical effects

Onset

Approximately 15 minutes after i.v. injection; 0.5–2 hours after ingestion.

Common signs

Drowsiness, vocalization, ataxia, hypersalivation, hypothermia and lethargy.

Other signs

Aggression, excitability, bradycardia and disorientation. Respiratory depression and coma are rare.

Treatment
- If appropriate, give activated charcoal (see Decontamination).
- Apomorphine should be avoided (it is also an opioid).
- Administration of naloxone if respiratory depression or coma occurs.
- Symptomatic and supportive care.

Prognosis

Favourable with supportive care.

Caffeine exposure in dogs

Description/Source

Widely available stimulant in tea, coffee and chocolate; also present in some over-the-counter analgesics, stimulant and weight loss preparations. **Note:** Chocolate-coated coffee beans pose a particular risk of toxicity (see Chocolate).

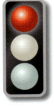

Toxicology

Caffeine is a methylxanthine structurally related to theophylline and theobromine. It acts as a stimulant on the central nervous system and muscles, including the myocardium. Methylxanthines inhibit cyclic nucleotide phosphodiesterases and antagonize the receptor-mediated action of adenosine. This results in cerebral cortical stimulation, myocardial contraction, smooth muscle contraction, and diuresis. Caffeine also stimulates the synthesis and release of catecholamines, particularly noradrenaline (norepinephrine). At high doses it stimulates the medullary, respiratory, vasomotor and vagal centres, but has less effect on cardiac stimulation and coronary artery dilation.

Risk factors

Cardiac disease.

Clinical effects

Onset

Usually 1 to 3 hours.

Common signs

Vomiting, diarrhoea, tachycardia, ataxia, tachypnoea, hyperthermia, diuresis, dilated pupils, polydipsia, hyperaesthesia, excitation, hyperactivity, irritability, restlessness, agitation, twitching and convulsions.

Other signs

Hypertension, cyanosis, coma and arrhythmias, particularly ventricular premature contractions.

Treatment

- Emesis is best avoided in hyperactive or excitable animals.
- Repeated doses of activated charcoal alone should be given (see Decontamination).
- Ensure adequate hydration and give anti-emetics if required.
- Diazepam can be used for hyperactivity or convulsions; if ineffective other drugs can be used (e.g. pentobarbital, phenobarbital, propofol).
- If possible, monitor the electrocardiogram.
- Propranolol may be useful for severe tachycardia or arrhythmias.
- Lidocaine can be used for ventricular premature contractions.
- Symptomatic and supportive care.

Prognosis

Favourable in dogs with mild stimulant effects. Guarded in dogs with severe stimulation or cardiac effects.

Calcium channel blocker exposure in dogs

Alternative names

Examples: amlodipine, diltiazem, felodipine, isradipine, lacidipine, lercanidipine, nicardipine, nifedipine, nimodipine, nisoldipine, verapamil

Description/Source

Used for the treatment of hypertension, arrhythmias and angina in humans. In dogs and cats they are used for hypertension, hypertrophic cardiomyopathy and tachyarrhythmias.

Toxicology

Calcium channel antagonists block L-type calcium channels. This blockade leads to vascular smooth muscle relaxation and negative chronotropic and inotropic effects.

Risk factors

None known.

Clinical effects

Onset

Usually within 6 hours, but may be delayed if a sustained release preparation has been ingested.

Common signs

Hypotension, bradycardia or reflex tachycardia, hyperglycaemia, lethargy and collapse.

Other signs

Convulsions, coma and pulmonary oedema.

Treatment

- Empty the stomach and give activated charcoal (see Decontamination). Repeat doses of activated charcoal may be given if a sustained release preparation is ingested.
- Check blood glucose.
- Intravenous fluids should be used initially for hypotension.
- Calcium borogluconate or calcium gluconate if unresponsive to intravenous fluids.
- Glucagon 50–150 micrograms/kg i.v. bolus could be considered in dogs unresponsive to calcium salts.
- Adrenaline can be considered if prior therapies have failed.
- Consider high dose insulin/dextrose therapy and/or intravenous lipid emulsion in severe cases.

Prognosis

Favourable in animals with mild to moderate effects. Guarded in animals with significant cardiovascular effects.

Cannabis sativa exposure in dogs

Alternative names

Marijuana, hash, weed, cannabis, pot, skunk

Description/Source

The plant is used to produce hemp (an industrial fibre). Hemp seed is eaten as a health food, and cannabis is used as a psychoactive drug.

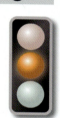

Toxicology

The main toxic constituent is delta-9-tetrahydrocannabinol (THC). This affects a variety of neurotransmitters including dopamine, serotonin and gamma-aminobutyric acid (GABA). Dogs may exhibit mild to moderate signs after passive inhalation but are more likely to become unwell after ingestion.

Risk factors

None known.

Clinical effects

Onset

Usually within 4 hours post ingestion or within minutes after inhalation.

Common signs

Ataxia, weakness, dilated pupils, vomiting, drowsiness, hyperaesthesia, urinary and faecal incontinence and behavioural changes.

Other signs

Bradycardia or tachycardia, hypotension, hyperthermia or hypothermia, tremors, twitching, muscle fasciculations and convulsions.

Treatment

- Empty the stomach and give repeat doses of activated charcoal (see Decontamination).
- Ensure adequate hydration and give anti-emetics if required.
- Symptomatic and supportive care.

Prognosis

Favourable.

Carbamate insecticide exposure in dogs

For exposure in cats – see page 123

Alternative names

Examples: aldicarb, bendiocarb, carbaryl, carbofuran, fenoxycarb, methiocarb, methomyl, oxamyl, thiodicarb

Description/Source

Carbamate insecticides are widely used as garden and household pesticides, and in agriculture. Formulations include liquids, sprays and powders which may be used as supplied or diluted. Domestic products usually contain a low concentration; agricultural products are more hazardous.

Toxicology

Carbamates act in a similar way to organophosphates, binding to and inhibiting acetylcholinesterase. This results in accumulation of the neurotransmitter acetylcholine and activation of nicotinic and muscarinic receptors. Therefore both nicotinic and muscarinic effects occur, although nicotinic receptors rapidly become desensitized. Effects resulting from carbamate poisoning tend to be of much shorter duration compared with those of organophosphate poisoning.

Risk factors

None known.

Clinical effects

Onset

Usually within 15 minutes to 3 hours.

Common signs

Hypersalivation, increased bronchial secretion, ataxia, diarrhoea, constricted pupils, muscle fasciculation, tremors, weakness, hyperaesthesia, hyperthermia and urinary incontinence.

Other signs

Collapse, bradycardia, respiratory depression, convulsions, cyanosis and coma may occur. Myopathy occurs rarely following recovery.

Treatment

- Empty the stomach and give activated charcoal (see Decontamination).
- Decontaminate the skin by washing with a mild detergent and lukewarm water (see Decontamination).
- Monitor body temperature and treat hyperthermia >41°C aggressively.
- Atropine should be given to reverse cholinergic effects.
- Use of a cholinesterase reactivator (such as pralidoxime) is unnecessary.
- Symptomatic and supportive care.

Prognosis

Favourable with aggressive supportive care.

Carbamazepine exposure in dogs

Description/Source

Anticonvulsant drug used in human medicine in all types of epilepsy, except absence seizures, and for trigeminal neuralgia. Tablet formulations are commonly sustained release preparations. Carbamazepine is no longer used for the treatment of epilepsy in dogs owing to rapid metabolism and a short half-life.

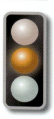

Toxicology

The mechanism of action of carbamazepine has not been fully elucidated. It stabilizes hyperexcited nerve membranes, inhibits repetitive neuronal discharges and reduces synaptic propagation of excitatory impulses.

Risk factors

None known.

Clinical effects

Onset

Usually 1 to 2 hours, but may be delayed if a sustained release preparation has been ingested.

Common signs

Drowsiness, lethargy, ataxia and vomiting.

Other signs

Twitching, muscle spasms and convulsions.

Treatment

- Empty the stomach and give activated charcoal (see Decontamination).
- Anticonvulsants if required.
- Symptomatic and supportive care.

Prognosis

Favourable.

Carbon monoxide exposure in dogs

Description/Source

A colourless, odourless, tasteless, non-irritating, flammable gas. It is formed when there is incomplete combustion of organic fuels. Many incidents of carbon monoxide poisoning are associated with the use of badly installed, poorly maintained or malfunctioning domestic combustion appliances using gas, oil or solid fuel, or the use of such appliances in inadequately ventilated areas.

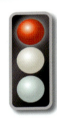

Toxicology

Carbon monoxide binds to the haemoglobin molecule, forming a stable compound. This results in impairment of oxyhaemoglobin formation and causes cellular hypoxia. The haemoglobin molecule undergoes a conformational change when carbon monoxide binds to a haem site, with a resulting increase in the affinity of the remaining haem groups for oxygen. The net result is a shift of the oxyhaemoglobin dissociation curve to the left, and a haemoglobin molecule that is poorly equipped to release oxygen to the tissues. Carboxyhaemoglobin can convert to haemoglobin again, but this takes time as the carboxyhaemoglobin molecule is so stable.

Risk factors

Elderly animals, cardiovascular or cerebrovascular disease or pregnancy.

Clinical effects

Onset

Variable, depending on the concentration and duration.

Common signs

Non-specific and variable clinical effects with vomiting, depression, tremor, drowsiness, lethargy, anorexia, tachycardia, tachypnoea and ataxia. Behavioural changes, deafness and blindness may occur. The mucous membranes may appear bright red or grey/cyanotic.

Other signs

Lactic acidosis, hypotension, convulsions, coma, arrhythmias and permanent neurological damage.

Treatment

- Remove from source.
- Administer 100% oxygen by endotracheal tube or tight-fitting mask.
- Monitor electrocardiogram if required.
- Ensure adequate hydration.
- Monitor blood gases if required but be careful with interpretation as P_aO_2 will be normal. Co-oximetry is required to assess severity of toxicity fully.
- Pulse oximetry is also affected by the presence of the carboxyhaemoglobin molecule and so is not useful for monitoring.
- Anticonvulsants if required.
- Symptomatic and supportive care.

Prognosis

Favourable if animal has mild effects. Guarded if animal has severe neurological effects.

Chocolate exposure in dogs

Description/Source

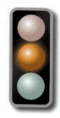

Confectionary containing theobromine, a methylxanthine, the major alkaloid in the plant *Theobroma cacao*. **Note:** Chocolate products may contain other toxic components such as raisins (see *Vitis vinifera* fruits), peanuts (see *Arachis hypogaea*) or coffee beans (see Caffeine).

Toxicology

Methylxanthines produce central nervous system stimulation by antagonizing cellular adenosine receptors. They also cause increased muscular contractility in both cardiac and skeletal muscle by inhibiting cellular calcium reuptake. The concentration of theobromine is higher in dark chocolate than in milk chocolate. White chocolate contains a very low concentration. Cocoa beans, cocoa powder and cocoa shell mulches contain the highest concentrations of theobromine.

Risk factors

None known.

Clinical effects

Onset
Generally within 2–4 hours, sometimes 6–12 hours.

Common signs
Vomiting, abdominal tenderness, hypersalivation, polydipsia, polyuria, excitability, tachycardia (sometimes bradycardia), ataxia and mild hypertension.

Other signs
Muscle rigidity, tremors, convulsions, tachypnoea, hyperthermia, cyanosis, arrhythmias and renal dysfunction.

Treatment
- If >14 g of milk chocolate/kg bodyweight or >3.5 g of dark chocolate/kg bodyweight has been ingested, empty the stomach and give repeat doses of activated charcoal (see Decontamination).
- Ensure adequate hydration and give anti-emetics if required.
- Sedation may be required.
- A beta-blocker (e.g. atenolol, propranolol) may be required for severe or prolonged tachycardia.
- Symptomatic and supportive care.

Prognosis
Favourable.

Codeine exposure in dogs

Description/Source
An opioid analgesic used for the treatment of mild to moderate pain, diarrhoea and cough suppression in dogs. The authorized canine preparation also contains paracetamol. Also available in some human over-the-counter preparations with paracetamol, ibuprofen and/or caffeine, and prescription preparations with paracetamol (co-codamol) or aspirin (co-codaprin).

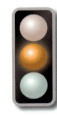

Toxicology
Codeine exerts its effects by binding to mu opioid receptors. Binding of codeine at the mu-1 receptors mediates the analgesic effects; binding at the mu-2 receptors is responsible for respiratory depression.

Risk factors
None known.

Clinical effects

Onset
Usually within 2 to 6 hours.

Common signs
Lethargy, drowsiness, vomiting, ataxia and constricted pupils.

Other signs
Respiratory depression, coma and hypothermia.

Treatment
- Empty the stomach and give activated charcoal (see Decontamination).
- Apomorphine should be used with caution.
- Naloxone should be given to those animals displaying signs of respiratory or central nervous system depression. Naloxone has a very short duration of action and repeated doses may be required.
- Warming measures if required.
- Symptomatic and supportive care.

Prognosis
Favourable with supportive care.

Colchicum autumnale exposure in dogs

Alternative names
Colchicum, autumn crocus, meadow saffron

Description/Source
Perennial flowering plant found in damp meadows and woods and widely cultivated. It flowers from May to October, before the leaves appear. The flowers are pink to lilac/purple or, rarely, white, and superficially resemble a crocus flower. The fruits ripen from April to August and are ovoid, green to brown capsules. This plant is different from and unrelated to the spring crocus (see *Crocus* species).

Toxicology
All parts of the plant are potentially toxic. The main toxic component is colchicine, an alkaloid amine. The greatest concentration is found in the seeds and the bulb. Colchicine has an anti-mitotic effect, which inhibits spindle formation in the metaphase stage of cell division and

therefore has most effect on cells with a high turnover rate (e.g. bone marrow cells, epithelial cells of the gastrointestinal tract).

Risk factors

None known.

Clinical effects

Onset

Within 48 hours.

Common signs

Severe gastrointestinal irritation, hyperthermia and renal impairment, elevated liver enzymes, leucopenia and bone marrow depression.

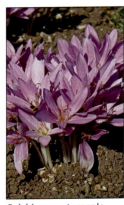

Colchicum autumnale.
©Elizabeth Dauncey

Other signs

Weakness, dehydration, recumbency, collapse and shock secondary to severe gastrointestinal irritation.

Treatment

- Empty the stomach and give activated charcoal (see Decontamination).
- Aggressive intravenous fluids.
- Gastric protectants are recommended (see BSAVA Formulary).
- Check haematology, hepatic and renal function.
- Any animal with evidence of bone marrow suppression should receive broad-spectrum antibiotic cover.
- Symptomatic and supportive care.

Prognosis

Guarded.

Cotoneaster species exposure in dogs

Description/Source

Evergreen low-growing shrub or tree commonly found in parks and gardens. They have small oval green leaves, white or pale pink flowers between May and August, and bright red berries from June/July onwards.

Toxicology

Although the bark, leaves, flowers and particularly the

fruit contain cyanogenic glycosides, the plant is considered to be of low toxicity.

Risk factors

None known.

Clinical effects

Onset

Within 4 to 6 hours.

Common signs

Hypersalivation, vomiting, diarrhoea which may be haemorrhagic, lethargy and ataxia.

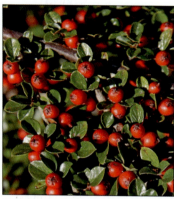

Cotoneaster horizontalis.
©Elizabeth Dauncey

Treatment

- Gut decontamination is not required.
- Ensure adequate hydration.
- Symptomatic and supportive care.

Prognosis

Favourable.

Crocus species exposure in dogs

Alternative name

Spring crocus

Description/Source

A widely cultivated and naturalized flowering corm (bulb). They have cup-shaped, solitary flowers that taper into a narrow tube. Flower colour is very variable, but lilac, mauve, yellow and white are common. The thin, grass-like leaf is green with a white central stripe. This plant is different from and unrelated to autumn crocus (see *Colchicum autumnale*).

Toxicology

Crocus is considered to be of low toxicity.

Risk factors

None known.

Clinical effects

Onset
Usually 2 to 4 hours, sometimes up to 12 hours.

Common signs
Anorexia, vomiting, diarrhoea and abdominal pain.

Other signs
Occasionally haematemesis and lethargy.

Treatment
- Gut decontamination is not required.
- Ensure adequate hydration.
- Symptomatic and supportive care.

Prognosis
Excellent.

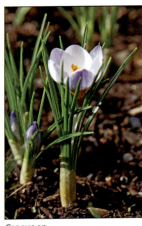

Crocus sp.
©Elizabeth Dauncey

Cyanoacrylate adhesive exposure in dogs

Alternative name
Superglue

Description/Source
Rapid-setting glue; also found in cosmetic nail adhesive.

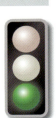

Toxicology
Cyanoacrylate glues are not toxic if ingested. On setting, heat may be produced and can cause local irritation. Most cases occur when the glue is applied to the ear or eye in mistake for ear or eye drops.

Risk factors
None known.

Clinical effects

Onset
Immediate.

Common signs

After ingestion: Local irritation, vomiting and hypersalivation. Risk of obstruction if large solid lumps are swallowed.

Eye exposure: Pain and irritation. Risk of corneal abrasion and the eyelids may become glued together.

Ear exposure: Pain, burning and ulceration of ear canal. Occlusion of the ear canal may result.

Treatment

After ingestion:
- Oral fluids may be given.
- Lumps of glue that are firmly stuck to the teeth or lining of the mouth should **not** be removed. Any loosened lumps of glue should be removed gently.

Eye:
- Irrigate the affected eye.
- Symptomatic and supportive care.

Ear:
- Irrigate the affected ear.
- Manual removal of the glue should be attempted but complete removal may take several days.

Prognosis

Excellent.

Detergent exposure in dogs

Alternative names

Amphoteric surfactants, anionic surfactants, non-ionic surfactants, cationic surfactants

Description/Source

Common constituents of many types of household cleaners. Cationic surfactants are usually found in disinfectants.

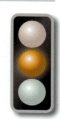

Toxicology

The effects of detergents are due to their irritancy. Systemic effects are uncommon. Cationic surfactants are more hazardous than the other types and can be corrosive.

Risk factors

None known.

Clinical effects

Onset

Usually within 12 hours, but will be more rapid following exposure to more concentrated solutions.

Common signs

After ingestion: Hypersalivation, vomiting, inappetence, diarrhoea and ulceration of the tongue and oral mucosa.

Skin exposure: Erythema, inflammation, hair loss and contact dermatitis. Concentrated solutions may cause chemical burns.

Other signs

With concentrated solutions or a cationic detergent there is risk of hyperthermia, respiratory effects, oesophageal ulceration and aspiration.

Treatment

- **Gut decontamination is not recommended.**
- If appropriate, decontaminate the skin by washing with lukewarm water (see Decontamination).
- Ensure adequate hydration and give anti-emetics if required.
- Analgesia if required.
- If there are respiratory signs, check lung sounds and perform chest radiography if required.
- Symptomatic and supportive care.
- Nutritional support may be required if oral ulceration is severe.

Prognosis

Favourable.

Dieffenbachia species exposure in dogs

Alternative names

Dumb cane, leopard lily

Description/Source

Popular houseplants. Can grow up to 2 metres but are usually smaller. The characteristically variegated leaves, usually 10 to 25 cm long, range from dark glossy green to pale green and yellow, white or silver.

Toxicology

All parts of the plant are poisonous; the main toxins are calcium oxalate and a proteolytic enzyme called dumbain. Water-insoluble calcium oxalate crystals are mechanically irritant and facilitate entry of other inflammatory or irritant substances into damaged tissue.

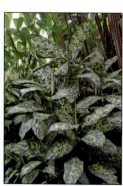

Dieffenbachia maculata.
©Elizabeth Dauncey

Risk factors
None known.

Clinical effects

Onset
Usually within 2 hours.

Common signs
Irritation and blistering of mucous membranes in the oropharynx, leading to hypersalivation, oedema and occasionally dysphagia. Vomiting, retching and diarrhoea.

Other signs
Severe oral ulceration and necrosis; oedema can result in airway obstruction and respiratory distress.

Treatment
- Gut decontamination is not required.
- Asymptomatic animals may be observed at home. Symptomatic animals should be seen and assessed.
- Ensure adequate hydration.
- Gastroprotectants (see BSAVA Formulary) and parenteral analgesia are recommended in symptomatic animals.
- Symptomatic and supportive care.
- Nutritional support may be required if oral ulceration is severe.

Prognosis
Favourable. Guarded in cases with severe oral ulceration.

Dihydrocodeine exposure in dogs

Description/Source
An opioid analgesic used for the treatment of moderate to severe pain in humans. Some preparations also contain paracetamol (co-dydramol).

Toxicology
Dihydrocodeine is an analogue of codeine, but is three times more physiologically active. Opiates exert their

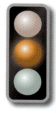

effects by binding to mu opioid receptors. Binding of dihydrocodeine at mu-1 receptors mediates the analgesic effects; binding at mu-2 receptors is responsible for respiratory depression.

Risk factors

None known.

Clinical effects

Onset

Usually within 6 hours, but may be delayed if a sustained release preparation has been ingested.

Common signs

Lethargy, drowsiness, vomiting, ataxia and constricted pupils.

Other signs

Respiratory depression, coma, bradycardia and hypothermia.

Treatment

- Empty the stomach and give activated charcoal (see Decontamination).
- Apomorphine should be used with caution.
- Naloxone should be given to those animals displaying signs of respiratory or central nervous system depression. Naloxone has a very short duration of action and repeated doses may be required.
- Warming measures if required.
- Symptomatic and supportive care.

Prognosis

Favourable with supportive care.

Diquat exposure in dogs

Alternative name

Diquat dibromide

Description/Source

A non-selective foliage-applied contact herbicide and desiccant.

Toxicology

In plants diquat acts by generating a superoxide ion, which damages cell membranes and cytoplasm. It is inactivated on contact with soil.

Toxicity is due to capacity for continual redox cycling. Diquat mediates protein oxidation (protein carbonyl formation) through multiple pathways, the precise mechanisms of which are unclear. It induces increased water secretion into the intestinal tract; it has been suggested from animal studies (rats) that this secretory effect is nerve-mediated and implies mast cell degranulation and nitrogen oxide release. Significant toxicity is far more likely with exposure to agricultural products (more concentrated) than with products for domestic use. Severe toxicity is uncommon in domestic animals.

Risk factors

None known.

Clinical effects

Onset

Up to 24 hours, but can be longer with agricultural products.

Common signs

After ingestion: Diarrhoea, vomiting and hypersalivation. Polydipsia, inappetence and abdominal discomfort in more severe cases.

Skin exposure: Domestic products may cause mild local irritation. Agricultural products may cause severe irritation, pain and chemical burns.

Other signs

With exposure to agricultural products: ulceration of mouth and gastrointestinal tract, oedema of oral mucosa, tongue and upper airway, with obstruction. Increased fluid secretion into gut lumen and ileus, renal failure, drowsiness, coma and cerebral oedema, mild elevations in liver enzymes, pancytopenia, bronchopneumonia and pulmonary oedema.

Treatment

- Gut decontamination is unlikely to be required after ingestion of a small quantity of a domestic product.
- Repeat doses of activated charcoal may be considered after ingestion of an agricultural product (see Decontamination).
- If appropriate, decontaminate the skin by washing with a mild detergent and lukewarm water (see Decontamination).
- Ensure adequate hydration and give anti-emetics if required. If an agricultural product is involved check hepatic and renal function, and haematology if concerned.
- Perform chest radiography if animal is dyspnoeic.
- Symptomatic and supportive care.
- In the case of severe oral irritation, nutritional support may be required through the use of feeding tubes.

Prognosis

Favourable.

Ethanol exposure in dogs

Alternative name

Alcohol

Description/Source

Ethanol has multiple uses. It is found in tinctures, elixirs, spirits (e.g. industrial methylated spirit is 95% ethanol), antiseptic preparations, mouthwashes, perfumes, aftershaves and colognes (where it may be present in concentrations up to 90%). Industrially it has uses as a solvent and sometimes as a fuel. Ethanol has some medicinal uses, particularly as an antidote in ethylene glycol poisoning. Most beers contain 3–6% ethanol by volume, wines 10–12% and distilled beverages (whisky, gin, vodka, etc.) between 20 and 60%.

Toxicology

Ethanol is a central nervous system depressant that is considered to act initially by depression of the reticular activating system. The exact mechanism is unclear but may involve interference with ion transport at the cell membrane.

Risk factors

None known.

Clinical effects

Onset

1 to 2 hours.

Common signs

Vomiting, diarrhoea, excitability and agitation, and then depression, ataxia, disorientation, vocalization and drowsiness.

Other signs

Coma, hypothermia, metabolic acidosis, hypoglycaemia, urinary incontinence and respiratory depression.

Treatment

- Empty the stomach (see Decontamination) if ingestion was very recent; absorption is extremely rapid.
- Activated charcoal is not useful.
- Ensure adequate hydration.
- Warming measures if required.
- Monitor and correct blood glucose if hypoglycaemic.
- If possible check blood gases/acid–base status.
- Symptomatic and supportive care.

Prognosis

Favourable.

Ethylene glycol exposure in dogs

For exposure in cats – see page 130

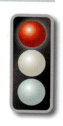

Alternative name

Ethanediol

Description/Source

Used widely as an antifreeze (often dyed a bright colour), in screen washes, brake fluid, inks, and as a coolant.

Toxicology

Ethylene glycol is converted by alcohol dehydrogenase to a number of toxic metabolites, and it is these compounds that are responsible for the renal damage and hypocalcaemia.

Risk factors

None known.

Clinical effects

Onset

Initial signs from 30 minutes to 12 hours.

Common signs

- Stage 1 (30 minutes to 12 hours): Depression, vomiting, ataxia, tachycardia, weakness, polyuria, polydipsia, hypocalcaemia and hypothermia.
- Stage 2 (12 to 24 hours): Cardiopulmonary signs with tachypnoea, acidosis, hyper- or hypotension, pulmonary oedema and arrhythmias.
- Stage 3 (24 to 72 hours): Renal signs with oliguria, azotaemia and renal failure.

Other signs

Oxaluria, hyperglycaemia, hyperkalaemia and hyperphosphataemia.

Treatment

- Gut decontamination is probably only worthwhile if the animal presents within 1 hour of ingestion (see Decontamination).
- Activated charcoal is not useful.
- Ethanol is a specific antidote and should be given as soon as possible. **Ethanol should not be given to dogs in renal failure.**
- Fomepizole, a competitive inhibitor of alcohol dehydrogenase, can be used; however it is expensive and not widely available.
- Sodium bicarbonate can be used for acidosis.

- Monitor renal function.
- Supportive care.

Prognosis

Favourable in animals with improving clinical signs within 24 hours of treatment. Poor in animals with renal failure.

Expanding foam exposure in dogs

Alternative name

Polyurethane foam

Description/Source

DIY or building product used as a gap filler, insulation or sealant. Usually available in aerosol cans (to be applied by hand) or in tubes (used in a hand-held gun applicator). A number of isocyanates are used (typically diphenylmethane diisocyanate, but also toluene diisocyanate or hexamethylene diisocyanate). The reaction of the diisocyanate and the urethane is exothermic, resulting in polymerization of the urethane and curing of the end product.

Toxicology

Systemic toxicity is not expected from ingestion of expanding foam. The risk is obstruction due to expansion of the foam in the stomach. Gastric foreign bodies only appear to have been reported with polyurethane adhesives containing diphenylmethane diisocyanate and not with other polyurethane expanding products, but there is a potential risk with expanding foam. Cured (i.e. set) foam is not toxic but may also cause obstruction.

Risk factors

None known.

Clinical effects

Onset

Variable, but often within 12 hours.

Common signs

After ingestion: Vomiting, haematemesis, anorexia, diarrhoea, lethargy, depression, abdominal discomfort and extension.

Topical exposure: The foam will set rapidly on the skin. Local irritation may occur.

Other signs

Mild gastric hyperaemia and ulceration; gastric perforation.

Treatment

After ingestion:

- **Gut decontamination is not recommended.**
- Oral fluids and food should **not** be given initially.
- Monitor for signs of gastrointestinal complications over the following 24 hours.
- Gastroprotectants are recommended (see BSAVA Formulary).
- Imaging may be required if gastric obstruction is suspected. Contrast imaging may be used to visualize obstruction in the stomach or intestines.
- Gastrotomy is required if gastric obstruction is suspected.

Topical exposure:

- Once set, the foam is very difficult to remove.
- Washing with detergent or vegetable oil may help; otherwise it is best to leave it.
- The coat may be clipped if necessary.

Prognosis

Favourable.

Fertilizer exposure in dogs

Alternative names

Plant food, NPK fertilizer, bonemeal

Description/Source

Used for gardening and agricultural purposes, there are a wide range of products available. Outdoor fertilizers may be in the form of granules, powder or liquid, whilst houseplant products are usually liquid. Most products commonly contain nitrogen, phosphorus and potassium (NPK fertilizers), although they may also contain trace elements such as iron. Note: Some fertilizers contain high concentrations of iron, and these are more toxic.

Toxicology

Fertilizers are generally of low toxicity. Clinical effects are thought to occur because of the irritant nature of the constituents.

Risk factors

None known.

Clinical effects

Onset
Usually 2 to 10 hours.

Common signs
Diarrhoea, vomiting, ataxia and borborygmi.

Other signs
Shivering, swelling of the muzzle, urticarial rash and transient hindleg stiffness.

Treatment
- Gut decontamination is not required.
- Ensure adequate hydration and give anti-emetics if required.
- Symptomatic and supportive care.

Prognosis
Excellent.

Fish oil exposure in dogs

Alternative names
Cod liver oil, halibut oil, salmon oil

Description/Source
Component of many human over-the-counter multimineral and multivitamin preparations.

Toxicology
These oils have low acute toxicity, even when ingested in bulk.

Risk factors
None known.

Clinical effects

Onset
Within 2 hours.

Common signs
Vomiting and diarrhoea.

Other signs
Dehydration.

Treatment
- Gut decontamination is not required.
- Ensure adequate hydration and give anti-emetics if required.

Prognosis
Excellent.

5-Fluorouracil exposure in dogs

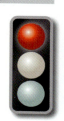

Alternative name
5-FU

Description/Source
An antimetabolite drug used in the treatment of cancer. It is also used topically for the treatment of pre-malignant and malignant skin lesions in humans.

Toxicology
A pyrimidine analogue that inhibits RNA processing/function and DNA synthesis/repair, thereby inhibiting cell division and causing cell death. Tissues with rapidly dividing cells (e.g. bone marrow, intestinal crypts) are most susceptible. Neurotoxicity is thought to occur because 5-fluorouracil is metabolized to fluorocitrate, which interferes with the Krebs cycle. Most cases in dogs are due to ingestion of human dermal preparations. Overdose results in gastrointestinal signs, neurological effects and then bone marrow suppression.

Risk factors
None known.

Clinical effects

Onset
Usually within 1 hour, sometimes up to 5 hours. Onset of bone marrow suppression is 4 to 7 days.

Common signs
Vomiting, ataxia, tremors, respiratory distress or depression and convulsions.

Other signs
Diarrhoea and gastrointestinal ulceration and haemorrhage, nystagmus, hallucinations, anxiety, hyperaesthesia, severe personality change, bradycardia or tachycardia, and cardiac arrhythmias. Bone marrow suppression is not commonly observed because most animals with severe fluorouracil poisoning do not survive.

Treatment

- Depending on the animal's clinical condition, empty the stomach and give activated charcoal (see Decontamination).
- If the exposure was dermal, the animal should be stabilized if necessary and then thoroughly washed with soap and water and dried.
- Ensure adequate hydration and give anti-emetics if required. Gastroprotectants should be given (see Ulcer-healing drugs in Formulary).
- Seizures can be refractory. Barbiturates, isoflurane or propofol can be given.
- Monitor blood count, liver and renal function.
- Blood transfusions may be required in animals with excessive blood loss.
- Any animal with evidence of bone marrow suppression should receive antibiotic cover because of the risk of infection. Filgrastim can be considered in these cases.

Prognosis

Poor in animals with signs of severe toxicity. Guarded in animals with only mild effects.

Fungus exposure in dogs

Alternative names

Mushrooms, toadstools

Description/Source

There are thousands of species of larger fungi in the UK. It is the reproductive part of the fungus (the fruiting body) that is visible and likely to be eaten. Identification is difficult without specialist knowledge and experience. If samples are collected for later identification they should be stored in paper (not plastic) and refrigerated. See also Puffballs.

Toxicology

Only a small number of fungi are poisonous, and effects depend on the type of toxin involved. Where toxic species are ingested, the sooner the onset of effects, the less toxic the fungus. If identification is impossible from a specimen, it may be possible to identify the syndrome of fungal poisoning from the clinical effects. In general, *rapid onset* of clinical effects (within 6 hours of ingestion) would suggest one of the following:

- Gastrointestinal irritant poisoning
- Ibotenic acid poisoning

- Muscarine poisoning
- Psilocybin poisoning.

Late onset of clinical effects (more than 6 hours after ingestion) would suggest one of the following:

- Amatoxin poisoning
- Gyromitrin poisoning
- Orellanine poisoning.

Risk factors

None known.

Clinical effects

Onset

Depends on the syndrome:
- Gastrointestinal irritants: 25 to 120 minutes
- Ibotenic acid: 30 to 120 minutes
- Muscarine: within 30 minutes
- Psilocybin: 10 to 30 minutes
- Amatoxins: 6 to 24 hours
- Gyromitrin: 2 to 24 hours; severe effects 36 to 48 hours
- Orellanine: Up to 17 days.

Common signs

Clinical effects from ingestion of fungi can be summarized according to syndrome:

- Gastrointestinal irritants: Vomiting, diarrhoea, abdominal tenderness
- Ibotenic acid: Vomiting, confusion and disorientation, ataxia, lethargy/hyperactivity cycles, hallucinations, twitching, convulsions and final phase of deep sleep
- Muscarine: Hypersalivation, lacrimation, constricted pupils, bradycardia, abdominal tenderness and watery diarrhoea
- Psilocybin: Dilated pupils, behavioural changes, tachycardia, hyperreflexia, vomiting and abdominal tenderness, depression, anxiety, hyperthermia and convulsions
- Amatoxins: Severe abdominal tenderness, vomiting, watery diarrhoea, dehydration, hepatic and renal failure
- Gyromitrin: Abdominal tenderness, vomiting, diarrhoea, lethargy, pyrexia, hepatic and renal failure
- Orellanine: Anorexia, vomiting, diarrhoea or constipation, polydipsia, polyuria and renal failure.

Treatment

- Depending on the animal's condition, empty the stomach and give activated charcoal (see Decontamination).

- Ensure adequate hydration and give anti-emetics if required.
- Ibotenic acid: A quiet, dark environment may be beneficial, with sedation if required.
- Muscarine: Atropine may be required.
- Psilocybin: A quiet, dark environment may be beneficial, with sedation if required.
- Amatoxins: Contact VPIS for specialist advice.
- Gyromitrin: Symptomatic and supportive, monitoring renal and liver function.
- Orellanine: Symptomatic and supportive care.

Prognosis

Excellent for most cases. Clinical effects starting within 6 hours of ingestion suggest a favourable prognosis. Guarded prognosis where a very toxic species has been ingested.

Gabapentin exposure in dogs

Description/Source

Gabapentin is an anticonvulsant and analgesic used in dogs and cats as adjunctive therapy for refractory or complex partial seizures, or the treatment of pain.

Toxicology

The precise mechanism of action of gabapentin is unknown. Although it is structurally related to the neurotransmitter gamma-aminobutyric acid (GABA), its mechanism of action is different from that of several other substances that interact with GABA synapses. Serious cases of gabapentin ingestion have not been reported in dogs.

Risk factors

None known.

Clinical effects

Onset

1 to 6 hours.

Common signs

Drowsiness, lethargy, depression, ataxia, disorientation, vomiting and diarrhoea.

Other signs

Respiratory depression, hypotension, tachycardia and convulsions.

Treatment

- Give activated charcoal (see Decontamination).
- Empty the stomach if required (see Decontamination).
- Symptomatic and supportive care.

Prognosis

Favourable.

Glucosamine exposure in dogs

Description/Source

Found in many joint supplement preparations, often combined with chondroitin, used in the management of osteoarthritis.

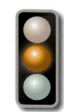

Toxicology

Most cases of acute ingestion of glucosamine joint supplements have minor or no clinical effects. However, there are reports of hepatic damage.

Risk factors

None known.

Clinical effects

Onset

Gastrointestinal signs usually 1 to 3 hours. Hepatic effects usually 24 to 48 hours.

Common signs

Watery diarrhoea, vomiting, abdominal tenderness and lethargy.

Other signs

Increase in alanine transaminase (ALT) and sometimes alkaline phosphatase (ALP) concentrations.

Treatment

- Gut decontamination is not required.
- Symptomatic and supportive care.
- Ensure adequate hydration.
- Check liver function of symptomatic animals, and use hepatoprotectant measures if indicated.

Prognosis

Excellent in most cases. Guarded in cases with elevated liver enzymes.

Glyphosate exposure in dogs

For exposure in cats – see page 134

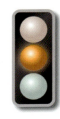

Description/Source

A broad-spectrum post-emergence herbicide; it is an organophosphate herbicide with no anticholinesterase activity.

Toxicology

The irritant surfactant, polyoxyethylene amine (POEA), present in many liquid preparations may be responsible for some of the effects reported. Some products contain up to 15% surfactant. The toxic mechanisms of glyphosate are unknown, but may be related to uncoupling of oxidative phosphorylation. Ingestion of treated plant material is likely to result in only mild gastrointestinal effects.

Risk factors

None known.

Clinical effects

Onset

30 minutes to 2 hours.

Common signs

Initially, gastric irritation (hypersalivation, vomiting, diarrhoea and inappetence), tachycardia and excitability, followed by ataxia, depression and bradycardia. Eye and skin irritation may occur.

Other signs

Collapse, severe bradycardia and convulsions. Rarely, pharyngitis, hyperthermia, twitching, dilated pupils, haematuria, renal failure and hepatic damage.

Treatment

- Empty the stomach and give activated charcoal (see Decontamination).
- Ensure adequate hydration and give anti-emetics if required.
- Check liver and renal function.
- Symptomatic and supportive care.

Prognosis

Favourable in most cases. Guarded in animals with renal or liver involvement.

Hedera helix exposure in dogs

Alternative names

Common ivy, English ivy

Description/Source

Native plant commonly found in woodlands, parks and gardens. Leaves are dark green with lighter green veins, often variegated with yellow. Small yellow-green flowers are produced from August to November; the fruits are small and black and arranged in clusters.

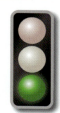

Toxicology

All parts of the plant are toxic, particularly the leaves and fruits. The leaves contain a saponin, which is irritant to mucous membranes. The allergenic compounds falcarinol and didehydrofalcarinol are also present.

Risk factors

None known.

Clinical effects

Onset

Within a few hours.

Common signs

Hypersalivation, vomiting, diarrhoea and abdominal pain.

Other signs

Allergic contact dermatitis.

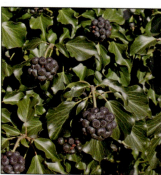

Hedera helix.
©Elizabeth Dauncey

Treatment

- Gut decontamination is not required.
- Ensure adequate hydration and give anti-emetics if required.
- Symptomatic and supportive care.

Prognosis

Excellent.

Hyacinthoides species exposure in dogs

Alternative names

Bluebells

Description/Source

Bulbous, perennial herbs native to woods, hedgerows and wet grassland throughout Britain and Ireland; also widely cultivated. The flowers are blue to violet-blue in colour and present from April to June. The fruits are ovoid capsules, containing 1 to 3 seeds and ripen from May to July. **Note:** Common bluebell (*Hyacinthoides non-scripta*), Spanish bluebell (*Hyacinthoides hispanica*), Italian bluebell (*Hyacinthoides italica*).

Toxicology

All parts of these plants (including the bulb) contain scillarens, which are cardiac glycosides similar in structure to those of the foxglove (*Digitalis* species). The cardiac glycosides found in plants are generally precursors that require enzymatic hydrolysis to produce the active glycosides. The gastrointestinal absorption of many primary glycosides is poor, and toxic concentrations are rarely reached following plant ingestion. Cardiac glycosides are negative chronotropes and positive inotropes. They cause decreased frequency and increased force of contraction of heart muscle. They also prevent outflow of sodium into the extracellular space, which increases the amount of calcium available for release during depolarization, increasing the force of contraction. Serious toxicity after ingestion of bluebells by dogs is rare.

Risk factors

None known.

Clinical effects

Onset

Within a few hours.

Common signs

Gastrointestinal and cardiac effects occur. Vomiting, diarrhoea (may be bloody), abdominal discomfort, lethargy, depression and bradycardia or tachycardia.

Other signs

Disorientation, hallucinations, hyperkalaemia, anuria and ECG changes.

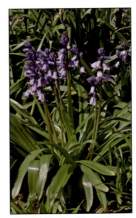

Hyacinthoides hispanica.
©Elizabeth Dauncey

Treatment

- An emetic is unlikely to be required unless a very large quantity has been ingested. Give activated charcoal (see Decontamination).
- Ensure adequate hydration.
- In a severe case check electrocardiogram and electrolytes.
- Bradyarrhythmias and AV block may require atropine.
- Ventricular tachyarrhythmias can be treated with lidocaine.

Prognosis

Excellent.

Hyacinthus orientalis exposure in dogs

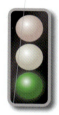

Alternative names

Hyacinth

Description/Source

A commonly grown house or garden plant. Bulbs are ovoid, about 6 to 8 cm across, with purple/white outer shiny papery scales. The leaves are usually glossy. Hyacinth flowers are pink, white, blue, purple or pale yellow and are strongly scented.

Toxicology

The plant contains various Amaryllidaceae alkaloids known to cause vomiting. The bulbs may contain up to 6% calcium oxalate, crystals of which are mechanical irritants. Oils from the plant cause dermatitis in humans.

Risk factors

None known.

Clinical effects

Onset

Within a few hours.

Common signs

Vomiting, retching, diarrhoea and lethargy.

Other signs

Abdominal distension.

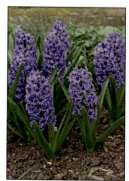

Hyacinthus orientalis.
©Elizabeth Dauncey

Treatment
- Gut decontamination is not required.
- Ensure adequate hydration.

Prognosis
Excellent.

5-Hydroxytryptophan exposure in dogs

Alternative name
5-HTP

Description/Source
An over-the-counter dietary supplement for depression. It is available in doses of 25 mg to 500 mg.

Toxicology
5-HTP is a serotonin precursor. It is rapidly absorbed and converted to serotonin (5-hydroxytryptamine, 5-HT). Serotonin excess results in overstimulation of serotonin receptors and produces central nervous system, gastrointestinal and neuromuscular effects. 'Serotonin syndrome' is a spectrum of clinical findings; not all are consistently seen.

Risk factors
None known.

Clinical effects

Onset
Within 10 minutes to 4 hours, with rapid progression.

Common signs
Behavioural changes and increased neuromuscular activity (ataxia, myoclonus, hyper-reflexia, shivering, tremor, nystagmus, hyperaesthesia) occur. Also, dilated pupils, hypersalivation, vomiting or diarrhoea, tachycardia and hypertension.

Other signs
Coma, muscular rigidity, hypertonicity, hyperpyrexia, metabolic acidosis, convulsions and acute renal failure.

Treatment

- Activated charcoal can be given depending on the animal's condition (see Decontamination); signs can progress rapidly and there is risk of aspiration.
- Treatment is supportive, with cooling measures as required and intravenous fluids to maintain hydration. Diazepam or phenobarbital can be used for agitation, tremors or convulsions.
- Cyproheptadine is a non-specific serotonin antagonist. *Dosage*: 1.1 mg/kg orally or rectally every 1 to 4 hours until signs resolve.
- *Phenothiazines, propranolol and metoclopramide should be avoided.*

Prognosis

Favourable with prompt aggressive treatment.

Ilex aquifolium exposure in dogs

Alternative name

Holly

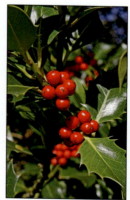

Description/Source

Common evergreen shrub with characteristic glossy, leathery, dark green leaves with spiky margins. The rounded fleshy berries (found only on female plants) are usually bright red, sometimes yellow or black, and grow in clusters. The plant is commonly available in the home as a Christmas decoration.

Toxicology

The leaves and berries contain irritant saponins that have local effects on mucous membranes. The leaves, berries and stems also contain cyanogenic glycosides. Severe poisoning in dogs is rare.

Risk factors

None known.

Clinical effects

Onset

Usually 2 to 3 hours.

Ilex aquifolium.
©Elizabeth Dauncey

Common signs

Vomiting, diarrhoea, hypersalivation, inappetence and depression.

Other signs
None.

Treatment
- Gut decontamination is not required.
- Ensure adequate hydration and give anti-emetics if required.
- Symptomatic and supportive care.

Prognosis
Excellent.

Iron exposure in dogs

Alternative names
Ferrous sulphate, ferrous fumarate, ferrous gluconate, ferric phosphate

Description/Source
Used in the treatment of iron deficiency. Iron salts are also a common constituent of lawn moss killers (which may be mixed with a fertilizer, e.g. lawn feed and weed).

Toxicology
Under normal conditions the amount of iron absorbed from the diet is determined by the body's iron requirement. There is no specific mechanism for the excretion of iron. Following an overdose the gastrointestinal barrier becomes overwhelmed and large amounts of iron rapidly enter the circulation. Unbound iron circulates freely, is distributed into cells and disrupts physiological mechanisms.

Risk factors
None known.

Clinical effects

Onset
Early effects within 6 hours. Late-onset effects after 24 hours. There may be a phase of apparent recovery between 6 and 24 hours.

Common signs
Initially, severe vomiting, diarrhoea, gastrointestinal haemorrhage and dehydration. Iron is radiopaque and therefore radiography may be used to confirm ingestion.

Other signs

Later, shock, coma, coagulopathy, liver and renal failure.

Treatment

- Empty the stomach (see Decontamination).
- Activated charcoal is not useful.
- Aggressive intravenous fluids with monitoring of renal and liver function.
- Administration of deferoxamine may be required.
- Symptomatic and supportive care.

Prognosis

Favourable in most cases with mild signs. Guarded where haemorrhage or shock has occurred.

Ivermectin exposure in dogs

Description/Source

Ivermectin is an avermectin antiparasitic drug used as an injection or spot-on formulation in dogs. Many cases of ivermectin poisoning in dogs occur from ingestion of equine products, usually spilled or dropped, or ingestion of manure from treated horses.

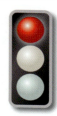

Toxicology

Avermectins are thought to act in mammals by potentiating the release and binding of gamma-aminobutyric acid (GABA)-gated chloride channels in the central nervous system. This results in cerebellar and cerebral cortex dysfunction. Collies and related breeds are more susceptible because changes in expression of P-glycoprotein allow increased uptake of ivermectin into the brain.

Risk factors

Collies, Australian Shepherds, Shetland Sheepdogs (also known as Shelties), Border Collies.

Clinical effects

Onset

Often within 3 to 6 hours but can be up to 12 hours.

Common signs

Ataxia, depression, hypersalivation, vomiting, dilated pupils, confusion and disorientation.

Other signs

Blindness (can occur in the absence of other severe clinical signs), tremors, convulsions, hyperaesthesia, hyper-reflexia, hypothermia or hyperthermia, weakness, coma and paralysis.

Treatment

- Empty the stomach and give repeat doses of activated charcoal (see Decontamination).
- Atropine has been used in the management of bradycardia.
- *Benzodiazepines and barbiturates should be avoided.*
- Propofol should be used for tremors or convulsions.
- Consider use of intravenous lipid emulsion in a severe case unresponsive to other therapies.
- Symptomatic and supportive care.

Prognosis

Favourable with good supportive care.

Laburnum anagyroides exposure in dogs

Alternative names

Bean tree, golden chain, golden rain

Description/Source

Laburnum is a cultivated ornamental tree, sometimes found growing on wild waste grounds. In summer, clusters of bright yellow flowers develop. Immature pods and seeds are green; ripe pods are pale brown, dry and contain 3 to 8 brown or black seeds.

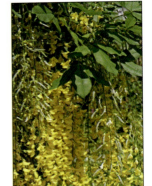

Toxicology

The main toxin is cytisine, a quinolizidine alkaloid, which is found in all parts of the plant. Cytisine has a nicotine-like action, although it has greater potency as a respiratory stimulant. It is rapidly absorbed. Severe cases of laburnum poisoning in dogs is rare.

Risk factors

None known.

Laburnum anagyroides.
©Elizabeth Dauncey

Clinical effects

Onset
Usually within 2 hours.

Common signs
Hypersalivation, persistent vomiting and diarrhoea.

Other signs
Lethargy, muscular spasms, incoordination and tonic-clonic convulsions. Death can result from respiratory paralysis.

Treatment
- Empty the stomach and give activated charcoal (see Decontamination).
- Ensure adequate hydration.
- Symptomatic and supportive care.

Prognosis
Favourable.

Lead exposure in dogs

Description/Source
Ubiquitous metal. Common sources are lead curtain and fishing weights, lead shot, lead flashing and lead paint.

Toxicology
Lead interferes with many enzyme systems, particularly those containing sulphydryl groups. This produces many effects, including impaired haem synthesis. The exact nature of the effect on the central nervous system is unknown, but probably involves interference with intracellular calcium function. The toxicity of lead compounds varies depending on their solubility.

Risk factors
Young age.

Clinical effects

Onset
Variable, depending on dose, duration, age of dog and existing body burden of lead.

Common signs

Anorexia, vomiting, colic, diarrhoea (or less commonly constipation), weight loss, hyperaesthesia, weakness, lethargy, behavioural changes, depression, head-pressing, tremor, twitching and intermittent seizures.

Other signs

Polyuria, polydipsia, nystagmus, blindness, ataxia, coma and megaoesophagus.

Treatment

- **Animals with gunshot wounds should be stabilized first; lead removal can be undertaken later, if necessary.**
- Radiography will confirm ingestion (or retention of gunshot pellets).
- If lead is present in the gastrointestinal tract a laxative is recommended.
- Monitor the blood lead concentration.
- Chelation therapy is recommended in animals with increased blood lead concentrations and/or signs of toxicity.
- In animals with signs of lead encephalopathy, treatment is supportive.

Prognosis

Favourable in asymptomatic animals. Guarded in animals with lead encephalopathy.

Levothyroxine exposure in dogs

Alternative names

T4, L-thyroxine

Description/Source

Levothyroxine is a naturally occurring thyroid hormone used for replacement therapy in thyroid-deficient states.

Toxicology

Thyroid hormone in **overdose** affects the cardiovascular, gastric and neurological systems. The effects may be delayed for several days during conversion of T4 to the active form T3 (tri-iodothyronine). A large dose is required before signs occur after an acute overdose, and toxicity is more likely from chronic overdosage.

Risk factors

Pre-existing cardiac disease.

Clinical effects

Onset

Can be 1–9 hours, but can be delayed for several days.

Common signs

Overdose (acute or chronic) results in a 'thyroid storm' with vomiting, diarrhoea, tachycardia, hyperactivity, agitation, irritability, lethargy, tachypnoea and dyspnoea.

Other signs

Polydipsia, polyuria, panting, pyrexia and hypertension.

Treatment

- Empty the stomach and give activated charcoal (see Decontamination).
- Propranolol can be used for tachycardia.
- Cooling measures and sedation, if required.
- Symptomatic and supportive care.

Prognosis

Excellent.

Loperamide exposure in dogs

Description/Source

A weak opioid with weak analgesic activity, used for non-specific chronic and acute diarrhoea.

Toxicology

At high doses, activation of opioid receptors in the central nervous system, together with increased circular contractions and decreased longitudinal contractions of the intestinal and colonic smooth muscle, are responsible for the toxic effects. Loperamide does not delay gastric emptying. Collies and related breeds are more susceptible because changes in expression of P-glycoprotein allow increased uptake of loperamide into the brain.

Risk factors

Collies, Australian Shepherds, Shetland Sheepdogs (also known as Shelties), Border Collies.

Clinical effects

Onset
Within 6 hours.

Common signs
Vomiting, depression, hypersalivation and drowsiness.

Other signs
Ataxia, abdominal tenderness, constipation, constricted pupils, vocalisation, bradycardia, dyspnoea, hypothermia, coma and collapse.

Treatment
- Apomorphine should be avoided (it is also an opioid).
- Activated charcoal is best avoided as it may exacerbate constipation.
- Ensure adequate hydration.
- In symptomatic cases monitor pulse, respiration and temperature.
- Administration of naloxone may be required.
- Consider use of intravenous lipid emulsion in a severe case unresponsive to other therapies.

Prognosis
Favourable.

Macadamia nut exposure in dogs

Description/Source

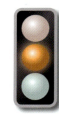

Macadamia nuts (from *Macadamia integrifolia* or *Macadamia tetraphylla*) have a very hard seed coat, enclosed in a green husk that splits open as the nut matures. They are eaten raw or in cakes and biscuits.

Toxicology

The mechanism of toxicity is unknown; it may involve a constituent of the nuts, processing contaminants or mycotoxins. Toxicity can also occur following ingestion of macadamia butter.

Risk factors

None known.

Clinical effects

Onset
Usually within 12 hours.

Common signs

Weakness and ataxia, abdominal tenderness, lethargy, vomiting, diarrhoea, depression, pyrexia, bloat, lameness, joint pain and recumbency.

Other signs

Mild increases in serum triglycerides and alkaline phosphatase.

Treatment

- Symptomatic and supportive care.
- Gut decontamination is not required.
- Ensure adequate hydration.
- Administer analgesic, if required.
- Check liver function, if required.

Prognosis

Excellent.

Mebeverine exposure in dogs

Description/Source

Antispasmodic used in humans for the treatment of irritable bowel syndrome and gastrointestinal spasm.

Toxicology

Mebeverine has a direct action on the smooth muscle of the gastrointestinal tract. It acts by reducing sodium ion permeability of smooth muscle cells and also indirectly reduces potassium ion efflux. It does not act through the autonomic nervous system and consequently has no anticholinergic effects.

Risk factors

None known.

Clinical effects

Onset

Within 3.5 hours.

Common signs

Vomiting, tachycardia, dilated pupils, drowsiness, ataxia, disorientation, excitability and convulsions.

Other signs

Hallucinations, hyperaesthesia and urinary frequency.

Treatment

- Empty the stomach and give activated charcoal (see Decontamination).
- Diazepam for excitability and convulsions.
- Symptomatic and supportive care.

Prognosis

Favourable.

Mefenamic acid exposure in dogs

Description/Source

A non-steroidal anti-inflammatory (fenamic acid derivative) drug used for the treatment of osteoarthritis in humans. Mefenamic acid is also used in humans for dysmenorrhoea and mild to moderate pain.

Toxicology

NSAIDs reversibly inhibit cyclo-oxygenase, thus blocking prostaglandin synthesis. Prostaglandins are believed to potentiate pain perception. Mefenamic acid is also irritant to the gastrointestinal mucosa. The mechanisms of toxicity are only partly understood. Unlike other NSAIDs, mefenamic acid causes convulsions; gastric ulceration and renal impairment are far less common.

Risk factors

None known.

Clinical effects

Onset

Usually within 1 hour.

Common signs

Vomiting, hypersalivation, tremor, ataxia, nystagmus, hyperaesthesia, tachycardia and convulsions.

Other signs

Restlessness, irritability, weakness, tachypnoea, collapse. Rarely, haematemesis and renal impairment.

Treatment

- Empty the stomach and give activated charcoal (see Decontamination).
- Ensure adequate hydration.

- Monitor renal function if required.
- Anticonvulsants if required (e.g. diazepam).
- Gastric protectants are recommended (see BSAVA Formulary).
- Symptomatic and supportive care.

Prognosis

Favourable with supportive care.

Metaldehyde exposure in dogs

For exposure in cats – see page 138

Description/Source

Metaldehyde is present in many molluscicide preparations. It is also found in fuel packs for camping stoves.

Toxicology

The mechanism of toxicity is not fully elucidated. It is suggested that toxicity results primarily from a decrease in inhibitory gamma-aminobutyric acid (GABA) concentrations.

Risk factors

None known.

Clinical effects

Onset

Extremely rapid, often within 30 minutes.

Common signs

Hyperaesthesia, muscle spasm and/or rigidity, tremors, twitching, convulsions, hyperthermia, panting, respiratory distress and cyanosis.

Other signs

Tachycardia, tachypnoea or respiratory depression. Liver damage can occur but is infrequent.

Treatment

- Owing to rapid onset of severe clinical signs induction of emesis is potentially hazardous, but in potentially severe cases gastric lavage under anaesthesia should be considered (see Decontamination).
- Twitching or convulsions need aggressive management, initially with diazepam but with escalation to full anaesthesia using propofol or isoflurane.

- Cooling measures may be required.
- Symptomatic and supportive care.

Prognosis

Favourable if mild signs occur. Poor if convulsions are uncontrolled.

Metformin exposure in dogs

Description/Source

Biguanide for the management of non-insulin dependent diabetes in humans.

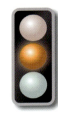

Toxicology

Metformin suppresses hepatic glucose production by decreasing hepatic glycogenolysis. Metformin does not tend to decrease blood glucose (it is antihyperglycaemic rather than hypoglycaemic).

Risk factors

Renal failure, chronic cardiac or pulmonary disease are risk factors for toxicity in humans and therefore presumably in animals.

Clinical effects

Onset

1 to 2 hours.

Common signs

Gastrointestinal irritation with vomiting, diarrhoea, lethargy and inappetence.

Other signs

Hypotension, hypothermia, pale mucous membranes and hindlimb tremors. In humans, lactic acidosis is the most significant effect seen in overdose, but this has not been reported in animals.

Treatment

- Empty the stomach and give activated charcoal (see Decontamination).
- Gastroprotectants are recommended (see BSAVA Formulary).
- Check electrolytes and blood gases if animal has signs other than gastrointestinal irritation or has renal impairment.
- Hypotension should be corrected with intravenous fluids. *Avoid fluids containing lactate (e.g. lactated Ringer's solution and diluents).*
- Acidosis should be corrected with sodium bicarbonate.

Prognosis

Excellent.

Methylphenidate exposure in dogs

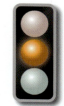

Description/Source

A central nervous stimulant used to treat attention deficit hyperactivity disorder (ADHD) in humans and narcolepsy and hyperactivity in dogs.

Toxicology

Methylphenidate is an indirect sympathomimetic; the mode of action is not fully understood but its pharmacological profile is similar to that of amphetamine.

Risk factors

None known.

Clinical effects

Onset

1 to 3 hours for normal release preparations, but may be delayed if a sustained release preparation has been ingested.

Common signs

Agitation, hyperactivity, pacing, ataxia, disorientation, hyperexcitability, tremor, tachycardia and hyperthermia.

Other signs

Lethargy and depression. Convulsions in severe cases.

Treatment

- Empty the stomach and give activated charcoal (see Decontamination).
- Symptomatic and supportive care.
- Acepromazine should be used for sedation if required.

Prognosis

Favourable.

Metronidazole exposure in dogs

Description/Source

Metronidazole is a nitroimidazole antibiotic for the treatment of infections with anaerobic bacteria, *Trichomonas* and *Giardia*. Also used in inflammatory bowel disease and hepatic encephalopathy.

Toxicology

The mechanism of toxicity is not known. The signs reported indicate cerebellar and central vestibular dysfunction, and metronidazole readily crosses the blood–brain barrier. The individual susceptibility to metronidazole is very variable.

Risk factors

None known.

Clinical effects

Onset

Within a few hours (acute); onset after chronic exposure can be very variable, usually days or weeks.

Common signs

Acute overdose is likely to cause lethargy, vomiting, anorexia and diarrhoea only. In **chronic exposure** there may be ataxia, weakness, inability to walk, nystagmus, disorientation, constricted pupils, tremor, hypermetria and head tilt.

Other signs

From **chronic exposure,** convulsions, coma, paresis, hypothermia, tachypnoea, hyporeflexia, extensor rigidity, opisthotonus, hyperexcitability and decreased proprioception.

Treatment

- **Acute overdose:** gastrointestinal decontamination and observation are unlikely to be required.
- **Chronic exposure:** treatment is supportive.
- Discontinue metronidazole.
- Diazepam is the drug of choice for metronidazole neurotoxicity and has been shown to improve recovery times in dogs.

Prognosis

Excellent.

Milbemycin exposure in dogs

For exposure in cats – see page 139

Description/Source

Milbemycin is a macrocyclic lactone anthelmintic, used alone or with other anthelmintics.

Toxicology

Milbemycin increases nematode and insect membrane permeability to chloride ions via glutamate-gated chloride ion channels. This leads to hyperpolarization of the neuromuscular membrane and flaccid paralysis and death of the parasite. Collies and related breeds are more susceptible because changes in expression of P-glycoprotein allow increased uptake of milbemycin into the brain.

Risk factors

Collies, Australian Shepherds, Shetland Sheepdogs (also known as Shelties), Border Collies.

Clinical effects

Onset

Within 6 hours.

Common signs

Anorexia, hypersalivation, vomiting, diarrhoea, dilated pupils, depression, tremor and ataxia.

Other signs

None.

Treatment

- Empty the stomach and give activated charcoal (see Decontamination).
- Consider use of intravenous lipid emulsion in a severe case unresponsive to other therapies.
- Symptomatic and supportive care.

Prognosis

Favourable.

Moxidectin exposure in dogs

Description/Source

Moxidectin is an antiparasitic drug structurally related to avermectins.

Toxicology

Moxidectin does not readily penetrate the blood–brain barrier in mammals, but can cause central nervous system effects at high doses. The cause of convulsions in moxidectin toxicity is unknown. Moxidectin is not inherently toxic to dogs but gross overdosage can cause signs of toxicity. This usually occurs when a dog ingests a preparation formulated for horses, as these are much stronger. Collies and related breeds are more susceptible because changes in expression of P-glycoprotein allow increased uptake of moxidectin into the brain.

Risk factors

Collies, Australian Shepherds, Shetland Sheepdog (also known as Shelties), Border Collies.

Clinical effects

Onset

Usually within 2 to 8 hours.

Common signs

Depression, hypersalivation, dilated pupils, ataxia, confusion, blindness, hallucinations, tremor, agitation, hyperaesthesia and hyperthemia.

Other signs

In severe cases, collapse, coma, twitching and convulsions.

Treatment

- Empty the stomach and give repeat doses of activated charcoal (see Decontamination).
- Atropine has been used in the management of bradycardia.
- *Benzodiazepines and barbiturates should be avoided.* Propofol should be used for tremors or convulsions.
- Consider use of intravenous lipid emulsion in a severe case unresponsive to other therapies.
- Symptomatic and supportive care.

Prognosis

Favourable with good supportive care.

Narcissus species exposure in dogs

Alternative name

Daffodil

Description/Source

Daffodils are perennial plants. They grow from a fleshy white bulb that is surrounded by a dark flaky skin. The daffodil is *Narcissus pseudonarcissus*, but there are many variants and hybrids. All *Narcissus* species have a central trumpet-shaped flower, typically yellow, orange or white. Double-flowered hybrids are available. The fruit is a small green capsule filled with minute black seeds.

Toxicology

Daffodils contain calcium oxalate crystals, alkaloids (particularly lycorine) and glycosides. These are present in all parts of the plant but are found in greatest concentration in the bulb. Alkaloids have irritant, emetic and purgative actions. Calcium oxalate acts as a mechanical irritant. Mild poisoning is possible if water in which cut specimens have been standing is drunk. Most cases of exposure occur in the spring when the plants flower or in autumn when the bulbs are planted.

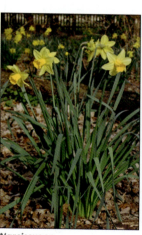

Narcissus sp.
©Elizabeth Dauncey

Risk factors

None known.

Clinical effects

Onset

Variable; from 15 minutes to 24 hours.

Common signs

Hypersalivation, vomiting and diarrhoea.

Other signs

Abdominal discomfort, lethargy, depression and hyperthermia. Rarely, dehydration, collapse, hypothermia, hypotension, bradycardia and hyperglycaemia.

Treatment
- Empty the stomach (see Decontamination).
- Ensure adequate hydration and give anti-emetics if required.
- Symptomatic and supportive care.

Prognosis
Excellent.

Nicotine exposure in dogs

Description/Source
Nicotine is an alkaloid from the tobacco plant (*Nicotiana* species). It is found in cigarettes, cigars, tobacco, snuff, electronic cigarettes and nicotine replacement therapy products. Note: Some nicotine replacement therapy products may also contain the sweetener xylitol.

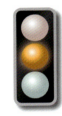

Toxicology
Nicotine causes cholinergic effects, with brief central nervous system stimulation followed by depression.

Risk factors
None known.

Clinical effects

Onset
Usually 15 to 90 minutes.

Common signs
Vomiting, hypersalivation, pale mucous membranes, ataxia, tremor, tachycardia, tachypnoea and hypertension, followed by bradycardia, respiratory depression and hypotension.

Other signs
Convulsions, coma and ventricular arrhythmias.

Treatment
- Empty the stomach and give activated charcoal (see Decontamination).
- Symptomatic and supportive care.

Prognosis
Favourable. Most cases involving electronic cigarettes develop only mild, if any, signs.

Nitenpyram exposure in dogs

For exposure in cats – see page 142

Description/Source

Nitenpyram is a neonicotinoid insecticide used orally in cats and dogs for the control of fleas.

Toxicology

Nitenpyram inhibits nicotinic acetylcholine receptors in insects but does not inhibit acetylcholinesterase. It is considered to be of low toxicity in mammals. Doses of up to 10 times the therapeutic dose have been well tolerated in dogs.

Risk factors

None known.

Clinical effects

Onset

1 to 2 hours.

Common signs

Increased scratching, hypersalivation, vomiting and diarrhoea. Malaise and shaking.

Other signs

Hyperactivity.

Treatment

- Gut decontamination is not required as severe effects are not expected.
- Symptomatic and supportive care.

Prognosis

Favourable.

Nitroscanate exposure in dogs

For exposure in cats – see page 143

Description/Source

Nitroscanate is an isothiocyanate anthelmintic used in dogs.

Toxicology

Nitroscanate is generally well tolerated, even up to 200 mg/kg. Effects do not appear to be dose-related and can occur at therapeutic doses or after a small overdose.

Risk factors

None known.

Clinical effects

Onset

1 to 12 hours.

Common signs

Ataxia, vomiting and lethargy.

Other signs

Weakness, elevated liver enzymes, inappetence, diarrhoea, tachycardia and head tilt may occur. Seizures and hyperthermia have been reported in a few cases.

Treatment

- Gut decontamination is probably not required unless a large dose has been ingested (see Decontamination).
- Symptomatic and supportive care.
- Check liver function if a large quantity has been ingested.

Prognosis

Favourable.

Non-steroidal anti-inflammatory drug (NSAID) exposure in dogs

These also affect cats – see page 144

Alternative names

Examples: aceclofenac, acemetacin, carprofen, celecoxib, dexibuprofen, dexketoprofen, diclofenac, etodolac, etoricoxib, fenbufen, flurbiprofen, ibuprofen, indometacin, ketoprofen, ketorolac, mavacoxib, meloxicam, nabumetone, naproxen, parecoxib, piroxicam, robenacoxib, sulindac, tiaprofenic acid, tolfenamic acid. See also Aspirin, Mefenamic acid and Paracetamol.

Description/Source

NSAIDs have both analgesic and anti-inflammatory effects, and are used in the treatment of pain associated with inflammation. NSAIDs reduce the production of prostaglandins by inhibition of cyclo-oxygenase enzymes. Prostaglandins are involved in control of gastric acid production, stimulation of secretion of mucous and bicarbonate by the gastric epithelium, and maintenance of mucosal blood flow. In the kidneys, prostaglandins take part in renal homeostasis. The isoform COX-1 is involved in the synthesis of regulatory prostaglandins, whereas COX-2 is inducible and is principally concerned with the synthesis of prostaglandins involved in the inflammatory response. Note: Some NSAID preparations contain the sweetener xylitol.

Toxicology

The toxicity of a particular NSAID depends on which isoform(s) of COX it inhibits, and to what extent.

Risk factors

Dehydration, hypotension, pre-existing renal insufficiency.

Clinical effects

Onset

Often within 2 hours.

Common signs

Nausea, vomiting, haematemesis, diarrhoea, melaena, abdominal tenderness and anorexia. Mucous membranes may be pale or congested. Also weakness, ataxia, incoordination, lethargy, depression and drowsiness. Gastric erosion, ulceration and, theoretically, perforation may occur in the absence of any other major clinical effects. Renal failure may be delayed for up to 5 days.

Other signs

Rarely, vocalization, agitation, hyperactivity, hyperaesthesia, tremors, twitching, dyspnoea, hyperventilation, tachycardia and convulsions.

Treatment

- Empty the stomach and give activated charcoal (see Decontamination).
- Aggressive intravenous fluids with monitoring of renal function.
- Give anti-emetics if required.
- Monitor renal function.
- Gastric protectants are recommended (see BSAVA Formulary).
- Use of prostaglandin analogue (misoprostol) is recommended.
- Symptomatic and supportive care.

Prognosis

Favourable if treated early. Guarded in animals with severe renal impairment or gastrointestinal perforation.

Oral contraceptive pill exposure in dogs

Alternative name

'The Pill'

Description/Source

Tablets may contain oestrogens and progesterone or progesterone only.

Toxicology

Oral contraceptives are considered to be of low acute toxicity.

Risk factors

None known.

Clinical effects

Onset

Within a few hours.

Common signs

Vomiting and diarrhoea may occur, but are not common.

Other signs

Progesterone-containing preparations may temporarily disrupt oestrus in bitches.

Treatment

No treatment is required.

Prognosis

Excellent.

Organophosphate insecticide exposure in dogs

For exposure in cats – see page 145

Alternative names

Examples: chlorfenvinphos, chlorpyrifos, demeton-*S*-methyl, dimpylate (diazinon), dichlorvos, dimethoate, fenitrothion, fenthion, heptenophos, malathion, pirimiphos-methyl

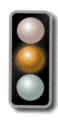

Description/Source

Garden, household and agricultural insecticides. Note some formulations contain petroleum distillate solvents.

Toxicology

Organophosphates (OPs) bind to and inhibit acetylcholinesterase, resulting in accumulation of the neurotransmitter acetylcholine and activation of nicotinic receptors. This results in both nicotinic and muscarinic effects, although nicotinic receptors rapidly become desensitized. OP insecticides are usually only present in low concentrations in domestic products and severe poisoning is uncommon. Agricultural products are more hazardous.

Risk factors

None known.

Clinical effects

Onset

Usually within 12 to 24 hours.

Common signs

Hypersalivation, ataxia, diarrhoea, constricted pupils, muscle fasciculation, tremors and twitching, weakness, shaking, hyperaesthesia, hyperthermia, restlessness and urinary incontinence.

Other signs

Bradycardia, respiratory depression, convulsions and coma. Some OP insecticides can cause delayed neuropathy.

Treatment

- Depending on the formulation, empty the stomach and give activated charcoal (see Decontamination).
- Decontaminate the skin by washing with a mild detergent and lukewarm water (see Decontamination).
- Atropine should be given to reverse cholinergic effects. Large doses may be required.
- Cooling measures if required.
- Pralidoxime may be given in severe cases. Pralidoxime is a cholinesterase reactivator, which dephosphorylates acetylcholinesterase. It is most effective when used as an adjunct to atropine therapy.
- Symptomatic and supportive care.

Prognosis

Favourable.

Paracetamol exposure in dogs

For exposure in cats – see page 148

Alternative name

Acetaminophen

Description/Source

A non-narcotic analgesic commonly found in combined oral analgesic preparations.

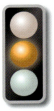

Toxicology

Paracetamol is metabolized in the liver by glucuronidation, sulphation and oxidation; the glucuronide and sulphate conjugates are non-toxic. The sulphation and glucuronidation pathways become saturated at high doses, resulting in more oxidation. This results in the formation of a highly reactive metabolite that depletes glutathione stores and then binds to cellular macromolecules to bring about cellular necrosis. In addition, metabolites induce methaemoglobin and Heinz body formation, and denature erythrocyte membranes.

Risk factors

- Malnourished state.
- Anorexia.
- Concurrent treatment with enzyme-inducing drugs.

Clinical effects

Onset

Within 4 to 12 hours; liver enzymes start to rise within 24 hours.

Common signs

Signs are due to hepatic necrosis and methaemoglobinaemia and include vomiting, depression, brown mucous membranes, tachycardia, tachypnoea, dyspnoea and hypothermia. Facial and paw oedema can be seen but are less common than in cats.

Other signs

Haemoglobinuria and renal failure.

Treatment

- Empty the stomach and give activated charcoal (see Decontamination).
- Acetylcysteine is an antidote that binds to toxic metabolites and acts as glutathione precursor.
- Monitor hepatic and renal function.
- Manage methaemoglobinaemia with vitamin C, sodium sulphate (1.6% solution; 50 mg/kg bodyweight i.v. q4h, up to 24 hours) and methylthioninium chloride (methylene blue) as required.
- Oxygen for respiratory distress.
- Symptomatic and supportive care.

Prognosis

Guarded; treatment with acetylcysteine is effective but prompt and aggressive management is essential.

Pergolide exposure in dogs

Description/Source

Dopamine agonist used in Parkinsonism, alone or as an adjunct to levodopa, in humans and used in veterinary medicine to control signs associated with equine Cushing's disease.

Toxicology

Pergolide is a dopamine receptor agonist that acts primarily on the D1 and D2 receptors. It stimulates striatal adenylate cyclase activity, which mimics the activity of dopamine.

Risk factors

None known.

Clinical effects

Onset

30 minutes to 2 hours.

Common signs

Vomiting, diarrhoea, lethargy and drowsiness.

Other signs

Ataxia, hallucinations and, rarely, hypotension and collapse.

Treatment

- Empty the stomach *if vomiting has not occurred* and give activated charcoal (see Decontamination).
- Ensure adequate hydration.
- Monitor blood pressure if required.
- Symptomatic and supportive care.

Prognosis

Favourable.

Phenothiazine exposure in dogs

Alternative names

Examples: acepromazine, alimemazine (trimeprazine), chlorpromazine, fluphenazine, levomepromazine (methotrimeprazine), pericyazine, perphenazine, prochlorperazine, promethazine, thioridazine, trifluoperazine

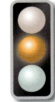

Description/Source

In animals phenothiazines are used for sedation and occasionally for the control of nausea and in the treatment of allergies. In humans they are used in the management of psychiatric disorders and in the control of nausea and vomiting.

Toxicology

Phenothiazine toxicity is variable; however, they all act on the central and autonomic nervous systems.

Risk factors

Giant breeds, boxers

Clinical effects

Onset

Within 8 hours.

Common signs

Lethargy, ataxia, drowsiness, bradycardia and occasionally excitability.

Other signs

Dilated pupils, hypotension, tremor and muscle fasciculation.

Treatment

- Empty the stomach and give activated charcoal (see Decontamination).
- Diazepam may be used for excitability or tremors.
- Symptomatic and supportive care.

Prognosis

Favourable.

Phenoxyacetic acid derivative herbicide exposure in dogs

Alternative names

Examples: 2,4-D, dichlorprop, MCPA, mecoprop and related compound, dicamba

Description/Source

Selective to broad-leaved plants, they are often used as lawn weed killers, combined with fertilizers and moss killers such as ferrous sulphate (see Iron). Also available in agricultural products. These chemicals are not very soluble in water, and solvents may be present in liquid formulations.

Toxicology

The mode of action of poisoning of phenoxy acid herbicides is not understood. The gastric effects are probably due to their acidity. They can damage plasma membranes, disrupt cell membrane transport systems and disrupt cellular metabolic pathways involving acetyl coenzyme A. They also uncouple oxidative phosphorylation, resulting in the energy that would be stored as ATP being dissipated as heat. In plants these compounds act as hormones; they have no hormonal action in animals. Severe poisoning with a domestic product is unlikely.

Risk factors

None known.

Clinical effects

Onset

Usually within a few hours.

Common signs

Vomiting and diarrhoea (may be haemorrhagic), lethargy, depression, hypersalivation, ataxia and anorexia.

Other signs

Collapse, weakness, bradycardia or tachycardia and tremor. Myotonia may occur.

Treatment

- Emesis is best avoided because of the risk of aspiration of the volatile solvents.
- Give activated charcoal (see Decontamination).
- If appropriate, decontaminate the skin by washing with a mild detergent and lukewarm water (see Decontamination).
- Ensure adequate hydration and give anti-emetics if required.
- Symptomatic and supportive care.

Prognosis

Favourable.

Pimobendan exposure in dogs

Description/Source

Pimobendan is a benzimidazole-pyridazone derivative used in dogs for congestive heart failure.

Toxicology

Pimobendan selectively inhibits phosphodiesterase III, resulting in increased intracellular cyclic adenosine monophosphate (cAMP) and vasodilation of peripheral and coronary vessels. It also increases the affinity of troponin C calcium-binding sites for calcium, which decreases the threshold for calcium-dependent myofibril contraction. Severe cases of overdose are rare.

Risk factors

None known.

Clinical effects

Onset

Within 4 hours.

Common signs

Vomiting, dizziness and hypotension. Tachycardia (after large doses).

Other signs

Ventricular extrasystoles, ventricular fibrillation, ventricular tachycardia, torsade de pointes. Increased liver enzymes and jaundice.

Treatment

- Empty the stomach and give activated charcoal (see Decontamination).
- Symptomatic and supportive care.
- Ensure adequate hydration.

Prognosis

Favourable.

Potassium bromide exposure in dogs

Description/Source

Potassium bromide is used in dogs for the treatment of epilepsy, alone or as an adjunct to phenobarbital. It is no longer used in humans in the UK.

Toxicology

Bromide displaces other halides in biological systems: chloride in the central nervous system and blood; and iodide in the thyroid.

Risk factors

None known.

Clinical effects

Onset

Bromide toxicity is subacute to chronic in onset, with a progressive course.

Common signs

Vomiting, diarrhoea, ataxia, incoordination, tremor and drowsiness.

Other signs

Quadriplegia and pseudohyperchloraemia.

Treatment

- In **acute** toxicity empty the stomach and give activated charcoal (see Decontamination). There is no benefit of gastric decontamination in chronic toxicity.
- Symptomatic and supportive care.
- Ensure adequate hydration.
- For severe toxicity, fluid therapy with 0.9% saline should be given to maintain hydration and encourage renal excretion by diuresis.
- Loop diuretics (e.g. furosemide) can also be used to enhance elimination.

Prognosis

Favourable.

Pot pourri exposure in dogs

Description/Source

A mixture of plant material (flowers, wood shavings, fruits, leaves, spices, fungi, lichen) used for scenting rooms. Hundreds of different plants are used. The scent is added using synthetic perfumes in refresher oils available separately.

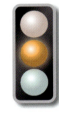

Toxicology

Pot pourri ingestion can result in significant, prolonged gastrointestinal signs. The reason for the long duration of effects is unclear. It may be due to physical damage to the gut rather than toxicity from the plant material or refresher oils. Effects have been reported to continue after the pot pourri has been passed in the faeces. Although toxic plants can be present in pot pourri this is uncommon.

Risk factors

None known.

Clinical effects

Onset

Usually within 12 hours; occasionally 24 to 48 hours after ingestion.

Common signs

Vomiting, anorexia and abdominal pain, depression, lethargy, ataxia, diarrhoea and dehydration.

Other signs

Hypersalivation, haemorrhagic diarrhoea, respiratory distress, collapse, convulsions and renal failure.

Treatment

- Gut decontamination is unlikely to be required as most dogs vomit anyway.
- Activated charcoal is not useful.
- Ensure adequate hydration and give anti-emetics if required.
- Gastroprotectants have been used in some cases.
- Analgesia may be needed.
- Symptomatic and supportive care.

Prognosis

Favourable.

Praziquantel exposure in dogs

For exposure in cats – see page 152

Description/Source

Praziquantel is a prazinoisoquinoline derivative broad-spectrum anthelmintic used in the treatment of trematode and cestode infections.

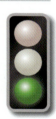

Toxicology

Praziquantel has a wide margin of safety and large doses have been tolerated in toxicity studies. The incidence of adverse effects in therapy is low. The mechanism of toxicity in mammals is unknown.

Risk factors

None known.

Clinical effects

Onset

Probably within a few hours.

Common signs

Vomiting, diarrhoea, hypersalivation, anorexia and lethargy.

Other signs

None.

Treatment

- Gut decontamination is not required.
- Symptomatic and supportive care, if required.

Prognosis

Excellent.

Proton-pump inhibitor exposure in dogs

Alternative names

Examples: esomeprazole, lansoprazole, omeprazole, pantoprazole, rabeprazole

Description/Source

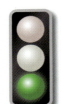

Proton-pump inhibitors are used for gastro-oesophageal reflux, gastric and duodenal ulcers and drug-associated ulceration in human medicine. Omeprazole is used in veterinary medicine to control gastric hyperacidity.

Toxicology

Proton-pump inhibitors inhibit gastric acid production by blocking the hydrogen–potassium adenosine triphosphatase (ATPase) enzyme system of gastric parietal cells. This results in potent, long-lasting inhibition of gastric acid secretion. These drugs are of low acute toxicity.

Risk factors

None known.

Clinical effects

Onset

Within a few hours.

Common signs

Rare and self-limiting. May cause vomiting, diarrhoea and lethargy.

Other signs

None.

Treatment

- Gut decontamination is not required.
- Symptomatic and supportive care.

Prognosis

Excellent.

Puffball exposure in dogs

Description/Source

Puffball is a general term referring to a number of fungi that release a fine cloud of brown spores when the mature fruiting body bursts. For toxic fungi see Fungi.

Toxicology

Puffballs are not toxic if ingested but the spores can cause respiratory signs if inhaled. The spores are hydrophobic and contain fungal allergens that can cause a hypersensitivity pneumonitis. The condition is sometimes called lycoperdonosis.

Risk factors

None known.

Clinical effects

Onset

Variable; it may be rapid or can develop over several days.

Common signs

Puffballs are not toxic by ingestion but may cause a mild gastrointestinal upset. Inhalation of puffball spores can cause lethargy, cough, sneezing, dyspnoea, tachypnoea, hyperthermia and leucocytosis.

Other signs

A chest X-ray may show bilateral infiltrates.

Treatment

- Gut decontamination is not required if ingested.
- For respiratory signs, supportive care with corticosteroids, antibiotics and oxygen if required.

Prognosis

Favourable.

Quercus species exposure in dogs

Alternative names

Oak, acorns

Description/Source

Oaks are large deciduous trees up to 45 metres high. The flowers are seen from April to May as the leaves appear. The fruits are green or brown acorns with cream-coloured flesh turning brown on exposure to air. Acorns ripen from August onwards.

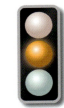

Toxicology

Quercus species contain tannic acid, but this may not be the only substance responsible for the toxic effects observed. The buds and immature acorns contain high concentrations of tannins. The effects are mainly gastrointestinal and renal. Tannic acid may lead to increased vascular permeability and subsequent vascular fluid loss, which may be the cause of oedema and tissue fluid accumulation (seen mainly in ruminants and horses). The individual response following ingestion of oak leaves or acorns is very variable. Some animals are severely affected; others not at all.

Risk factors

None known.

Clinical effects

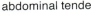

Acorns (from *Quercus* sp.).
©Elizabeth Dauncey

Onset

Variable; 1 to 24 hours.

Common signs

Retching, vomiting, diarrhoea, abdominal tenderness, lethargy and depression.

Other signs

Melaena, haematemesis, shaking, urticaria and gastrointestinal obstruction. Renal and liver damage are rare in dogs.

Treatment

- Empty the stomach and give activated charcoal (see Decontamination).
- Ensure adequate hydration and give anti-emetics if required.
- Check liver and renal function, if required.
- Symptomatic and supportive care.

Prognosis

Favourable in most cases. Guarded in animals with renal or liver involvement.

Quinine exposure in dogs

Description/Source

Alkaloid obtained from the bark of the *Cinchona* tree, used in human medicine for the treatment of night cramps and *Plasmodium falciparum* malaria.

Toxicology

Quinine is a stereoisomer of quinidine, and can cause myocardial depression and peripheral vasodilation. It also causes electrophysiological effects, such as an increase in action potential duration and effective refractory period and a decrease in membrane responsiveness, as well as a membrane-stabilizing, anticholinergic and alpha-adrenergic blocking action. Quinine can cause impairment of vision but the exact mechanism has not been elucidated.

Risk factors

None known.

Clinical effects

Onset

Usually 15 minutes to 2 hours.

Common signs

Vomiting, diarrhoea, lethargy, ataxia, tachycardia, hypotension, dilated pupils, transient deafness, hypokalaemia, hyperaesthesia and tremors.

Other signs

Blindness, collapse, convulsions, respiratory depression, cyanosis and arrhythmias.

Treatment

- Empty the stomach and give activated charcoal (see Decontamination).
- Ensure adequate hydration.
- Monitor electrocardiogram if possible.
- Electrolytes should be checked and corrected; avoid over-correction of hypokalaemia.
- Diazepam for convulsions.
- Intravenous fluids for hypotension.
- Sodium bicarbonate can be given for quinine-induced arrhythmias. *Avoid lidocaine, quinidine and procainamide.*

Prognosis

Favourable with supportive care. Guarded if severe cardiac effects.

Rhododendron species exposure in dogs

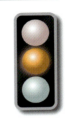

Alternative names

Rhododendron, azalea

Description/Source

Hardy, evergreen or deciduous shrubs and trees, commonly found outdoors and as house and conservatory plants. Flowers are either bell- or funnel-shaped and borne in clusters, and range in colour from white through red, pink and purple.

Toxicology

All parts of the plant are toxic and contain several diterpene resinoids called grayanotoxins. These compounds bind to receptors of the open and closed sodium channel of cell membranes, resulting in a modified sodium channel that undergoes slow opening.

Risk factors

None known.

Clinical effects

Onset

Within 20 minutes to 2 hours.

Common signs

Hypersalivation, vomiting, diarrhoea, inappetence, abdominal tenderness, trembling, staggering, lethargy, weakness, bradycardia, hypotension and exhaustion.

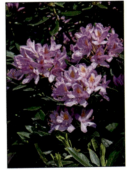

Rhododendron sp.
©Elizabeth Dauncey

Other signs

Fatal cases are very rare in dogs and are due to respiratory failure.

Treatment

- Empty the stomach and give activated charcoal (see Decontamination).
- Ensure adequate hydration and give anti-emetics if required.
- Atropine is a partial antagonist of the cardiac effects of grayanotoxins and may be considered if the animal develops severe bradycardia.
- Symptomatic and supportive care.

Prognosis

Favourable.

Salbutamol exposure in dogs

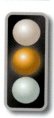

Alternative name

Albuterol

Description/Source

Salbutamol is a selective beta-2 agonist used in the treatment of asthma and other conditions associated with reversible airway obstruction in humans. It is available as tablets or an oral solution, and in inhalation devices.

Toxicology

Although salbutamol is a selective beta-2 agonist, this specificity is lost at high doses. Beta-1 receptor activation results in positive chronotropic and inotropic effects on the heart and beta-2 receptors in skeletal muscle are overstimulated.

Risk factors

- Pre-existing tachyarrhythmia.
- Cardiac insufficiency.

Clinical effects

Onset

30 minutes to 12 hours; commonly within 4 hours.

Common signs

Tachycardia, tachypnoea, vomiting, lethargy, panting, hypokalaemia and tremor.

Other signs

Restlessness, polydipsia, weakness, hyperaesthesia, dilated pupils and peripheral vasodilation.

Treatment

- After ingestion, empty the stomach and give activated charcoal (see Decontamination).
- Gut decontamination is not required if an inhaler has been punctured.
- Check electrolytes (especially potassium); monitor pulse, respiration and temperature.
- A beta-blocker (e.g. propranolol, atenolol) is recommended for hypokalaemia and may be required for severe or prolonged tachycardia.
- Symptomatic and supportive care.

Prognosis

Favourable.

Selective serotonin re-uptake inhibitor (SSRI) antidepressant exposure in dogs

Alternative names

Examples: citalopram, dapoxetine, escitalopram, fluoxetine, fluvoxamine, paroxetine, sertraline

Description/Source

Antidepressants; dapoxetine is used for premature ejaculation in humans. Also used for behavioural disorders in animals.

Toxicology

These drugs are selective serotonin reuptake inhibitors (SSRIs) and they have no, or minimal, effect on uptake of noradrenaline (NA), dopamine (DA) or gamma-aminobutyric acid (GABA).

Risk factors

None known.

Clinical effects

Onset
Usually within 4 hours.

Common signs
Drowsiness and lethargy; sometimes hyperactivity and excitability.

Other signs
Vomiting, restlessness, tachycardia, tremor and dilated pupils. Convulsions are rare. Risk of serotonin syndrome.

Treatment
- Empty the stomach and give activated charcoal (see Decontamination).
- Diazepam for convulsions or prolonged tachycardia.
- Symptomatic and supportive care.
- Cyproheptadine is the treatment of choice for serotonin syndrome. *Dosage:* 1.1 mg/kg orally or rectally every 1 to 4 hours until signs resolve.

Prognosis

Excellent.

Senna exposure in dogs

Description/Source

Plant-derived laxative used in humans and available over the counter. **Note:** some products are chocolate-based (see Chocolate).

Toxicology

Senna is metabolized by microorganisms in the large intestine to pharmacologically active compounds that reduce gut motility. There is reduced gut transit time and prevention of colonic water absorption, producing frequent watery faeces. The individual response is very variable.

Risk factors

None known.

Clinical effects

Onset

Usually 6 to 12 hours.

Common signs

Diarrhoea, vomiting and abdominal discomfort.

Other signs

Severe fluid loss may cause electrolyte imbalance.

Treatment

- Gut decontamination is not required.
- Allow access to drinking water.
- In severe cases intravenous fluids may be required.
- Symptomatic and supportive care.

Prognosis

Excellent.

Silica gel exposure in dogs

Description/Source

Silica gel is a commonly used desiccant and is often present in small packets in the packaging of electrical goods, shoes, cameras and containers for drugs.

Toxicology

Silica gel is inert and not toxic. Although packets are often labelled with a skull and cross bones and Do not eat, this warning relates to the substance being a non-food item.

Risk factors

None known.

Clinical effects

Onset
Not applicable.

Common signs
None anticipated.

Other signs
None anticipated.

Treatment

No treatment required.

Prognosis

Excellent.

Sodium chloride exposure in dogs

Alternative names

Salt, including salt water emetic, table or cooking salt, dishwasher salt, rock salt and seawater

Description/Source

Widely available and has many uses. It occurs as a white crystalline powder or colourless crystals and is found in bottle-sterilizing fluids, water softeners, some bath products (e.g. bath salts) and many foods (e.g. stock cubes, gravy products). It is also used in homemade dough for modelling. Iatrogenic toxicity is also possible following inappropriate use of hypertonic fluid preparations.

Toxicology

Sodium contributes to about 90% of the osmolality of the extracellular fluid, and an increase in sodium will increase the plasma osmolality. This results in the extracellular fluid becoming hypertonic, and in water moving from the intracellular to the extracellular space. The net result is cellular dehydration and vascular overload. In the central nervous system this causes vascular stasis, thrombosis, brain shrinkage and shearing of intracerebral vessels, with subsequent haemorrhage. Signs of toxicity are expected after ingestion of 2 to 3 g of sodium chloride/kg bodyweight and ingestion of 4 g/kg is considered lethal. Signs of hypernatraemia typically occur with acute increases of serum sodium concentrations above 170 mmol/l, with serious signs above 180 mmol/l.

Risk factors

Renal impairment.

Clinical effects

Onset

Vomiting can occur within a few minutes. Neurological signs can develop within an hour (in severe cases) or several hours later.

Common signs

Initial signs of hypernatraemia are non-specific, with vomiting, diarrhoea, depression, lethargy, tremor, polydipsia, dehydration, ataxia, weakness, hypertension, tachycardia and tachypnoea. Neurological signs progress to convulsions, coma and death in severe cases.

Other signs

Muscular rigidity, hyperchloraemia and mixed metabolic and respiratory acidosis, renal failure and electrocardiogram changes (including prolonged QT interval). Severe disruption to intracellular processes may occur due to severe intracellular fluid loss.

Treatment

- Empty the stomach (see Decontamination).
- Activated charcoal is not useful.
- Monitor electrolytes (particularly sodium concentration), blood glucose, blood pH, renal function and urine output. Monitoring of intravascular volume and hydration status is essential.

- The aim of treatment is to replace water and electrolytes and to aid renal excretion of sodium.
- In mild cases the animal should be allowed to drink small amounts of fresh water at frequent intervals.
- In most patients with **hypernatraemia**, the hypernatraemia has developed slowly (over days to weeks) and it is essential that the sodium and osmolality is not corrected too rapidly. Ideally the sodium should be corrected no faster than 0.5 mmol/l/h (or 10 to 12 mmol/l/day). Rapid reduction of sodium concentration can cause movement of water into the brain and result in cerebral oedema and convulsions. With **very chronic hypernatraemia**, sodium correction should be even slower (over 48 to 72 hours). However, in some rare cases (often acute ingestion) where the clinician is confident that the hypernatraemia has developed very rapidly (over hours) it is appropriate to correct the serum sodium over the same timeframe over which it developed.
- Fluid therapy will be influenced by a number of factors, including the animal's hydration state, renal function, haemodynamic status and, most importantly, serial measurement of serum sodium.
- If there is renal impairment and risk of fluid overload a loop diuretic (e.g. furosemide) should be used in addition to fluid therapy.

Prognosis

Favourable in mild cases. Guarded in dogs with neurological effects.

Sodium hypochlorite exposure in dogs

Alternative name

Bleach (chlorine-based)

Description/Source

A general disinfectant and bleaching agent.

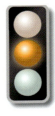

Toxicology

Sodium hypochlorite solution causes mucosal irritation, the extent of which depends on the volume ingested, the viscosity and concentration of the preparation and the duration of contact. Although sodium hypochlorite solution is alkaline it does not tend to cause corrosive damage except following ingestion of a large quantity or a concentrated solution. Severe effects from ingestion of a small quantity of household bleach are unlikely.

Risk factors

None known.

Clinical effects

Onset
Usually within 6 hours, some effects may be delayed by up to 24 hours.

Common signs
Hypersalivation, vomiting, lethargy and inappetence.

Other signs
Oral and tongue ulceration, diarrhoea, polydipsia, haematemesis, collapse, dysphagia, hyperthermia or hypothermia, respiratory distress and convulsions. Hypernatraemia, hyperchloraemic acidosis and increased serum osmolality. May cause mild local irritation on topical exposure (depending on the concentration).

Treatment
- Encourage oral fluid intake (milk or water).
- Ensure adequate hydration and give anti-emetics if required.
- In animals with signs other that gastrointestinal effects or where the quantity ingested is large, check electrolytes and blood gases.
- Symptomatic and supportive care.

Prognosis
Favourable.

Sodium valproate exposure in dogs

Description/Source
Sodium valproate is an anti-epileptic drug used in all forms of epilepsy and for migraine prophylaxis in humans.

Toxicology
Thought to act by inhibition of gamma-aminobutyric acid (GABA) transaminase, therefore resulting in an increase of GABA. Also inhibits voltage-gated sodium channels.

Risk factors
None known.

Clinical effects

Onset
Typically within 1 to 3 hours.

Common signs

Vomiting, ataxia, lethargy, drowsiness, hyperactivity and tremor.

Other signs

None.

Treatment

- Empty the stomach and give activated charcoal (see Decontamination).
- Symptomatic and supportive care.

Prognosis

Favourable.

Solanum tuberosum exposure in dogs

Alternative name

Potato

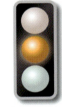

Description/Source

Annual plant growing up to 80 cm, with underground rhizomes that become swollen at the tip to form the tubers (potatoes); of major agricultural importance and also widely cultivated.

Toxicology

Solanum tuberosum contains the glycoalkaloids alpha-solanine and alpha-chaconine. These can cause gastrointestinal system effects due to membrane disruption. Fatal poisoning in animals is rare.

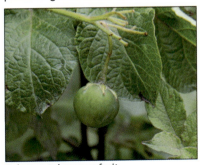

Solanum tuberosum fruit.
©Elizabeth Dauncey

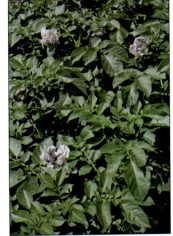

Solanum tuberosum flower.
©Elizabeth Dauncey

Risk factors

None known.

Clinical effects

Onset

Hypersalivation, vomiting, diarrhoea, inappetence, lethargy and ataxia. May be delayed 12 hours or more.

Common signs

Vomiting, diarrhoea (may be bloody), abdominal pain, ataxia, anorexia and lethargy.

Other signs

Hypothermia, melaena, haematemesis, haematuria and collapse. Risk of oesophageal or gastrointestinal obstruction if large pieces are swallowed.

Treatment

- Ingestion of ripe potatoes does not merit intervention.
- Gut decontamination is generally not required as it occurs spontaneously.
- Ensure adequate hydration and give anti-emetics if required.
- Symptomatic and supportive care.

Prognosis

Excellent.

Sorbus aucuparia exposure in dogs

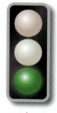

Alternative names

Rowan, mountain ash

Description/Source

A deciduous tree commonly found throughout the UK. It flowers from May to June with a creamy blossom. The berries are orange-red (sometimes yellow), and develop and ripen from August onwards, remaining on the plant to December.

Toxicology

The plant contains the cyanogenic glycoside amygdalin, and also parascorbic acid, which is irritant to mucous membranes. These compounds are present in very low concentrations and therefore rarely cause more than gastrointestinal effects.

Risk factors

None known.

Clinical effects

Onset

Often within 8 hours, but may be delayed up to 24 hours.

Common signs

Vomiting, diarrhoea and hypersalivation.

Other signs

Haemorrhagic diarrhoea.

Treatment

- Gut decontamination is not required.
- Symptomatic and supportive care.

Prognosis

Favourable.

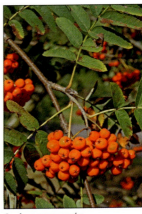

Sorbus aucuparia.
©Elizabeth Dauncey

Spinosad exposure in dogs

Alternative names

Spinosyn A, spinosyn D

Description/Source

Insecticide used in some fly and ant killers (usually in low concentrations). Also used orally for the control of fleas in cats and dogs.

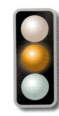

Toxicology

In insects spinosad activates nicotinic acetylcholine receptors. There is limited evidence to suggest that use in pregnant animals may be associated with adverse events. Spinosad is concentrated in milk. Animals receiving spinosad with high-dose 'off-label' ivermectin are at risk of ivermectin toxicity.

Risk factors

Epilepsy, possibly suckling young whose mother has been exposed.

Clinical effects

Onset

1 hour.

Common signs

Vomiting, inappetence, diarrhoea, polydipsia, lethargy or hyperactivity and vocalizing.

Other signs

Convulsions may occur in dogs with epilepsy.

Treatment

- Gut decontamination is not required, except in epileptic animals.
- In epileptic dogs empty the stomach and give activated charcoal (see Decontamination).
- Symptomatic and supportive care.

Prognosis

Excellent. Favourable in epileptic animals.

Statins exposure in dogs

Alternative names

HMG-CoA (3-hydroxy-3-methylglutaryl-Coenzyme A) reductase inhibitors. Examples: atorvastatin, fluvastatin, pravastatin, rosuvastatin, simvastatin

Description/Source

Statins are drugs used for the treatment of hypercholesterolaemia in humans.

Toxicology

Statins inhibit HMG-CoA reductase, an enzyme involved in cholesterol synthesis. Statins are of low toxicity to dogs following acute exposure. Most dogs show no clinical effects.

Risk factors

None known.

Clinical effects

Onset

Within a few hours.

Common signs

Effects are unlikely following acute overdose but vomiting, diarrhoea and abdominal tenderness are possible.

Other signs

None from acute ingestion.

Treatment

- Gut decontamination is not required.
- Symptomatic and supportive care.

Prognosis

Excellent.

Sulphonylurea exposure in dogs

Alternative names

Examples: chlorpropamide, glibenclamide (glyburide), gliclazide, glimepiride, glipizide, tolbutamide

Description/Source

Used in humans to lower blood glucose in non-insulin-dependent diabetes.

Toxicology

Sulphonylureas directly stimulate the acute release of insulin from functioning beta cells of pancreatic islet tissue, thereby lowering blood glucose.

Risk factors

None known.

Clinical effects

Onset

Variable and unpredictable; can be up to 24 hours.

Common signs

Hypoglycaemia with vomiting, abdominal discomfort, agitation and tachycardia.

Other signs

Coma, hypokalaemia, convulsions, metabolic acidosis, cerebral oedema, hypotension and cardiovascular collapse.

Treatment

- Empty the stomach and give activated charcoal (see Decontamination).

- Ensure adequate hydration.
- Monitor blood glucose and electrolytes frequently.
- Administer intravenous glucose (dextrose) if required.
- Symptomatic and supportive care.

Prognosis

Favourable with supportive care.

Sympathomimetic exposure in dogs

Alternative names

Examples: ephedrine, norpseudoephedrine, phenylephrine, phenylpropanolamine, pseudoephedrine

Description/Source

Used as decongestants and for sphincter hypotonus in cats and dogs. Used as decongestants and slimming aids in human medicine.

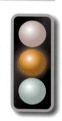

Toxicology

Sympathomimetics have direct and indirect effects on adrenergic receptors, and toxicity is due to acute cardiovascular and central stimulant effects. This results in endogenous release of catecholamines in the heart and brain, causing peripheral vasoconstriction, cardiac stimulation and increased blood pressure. Individual response is very variable.

Risk factors

None known.

Clinical effects

Onset

30 minutes to 8 hours.

Common signs

Stimulation, with tachycardia, agitation, hyperactivity, panting, hyperthermia and hypertension or rebound hypotension, dilated pupils and hallucinations.

Other signs

In severe cases bradycardia, tremors and convulsions. Risk of disseminated intravascular coagulation or rhabdomyolysis, renal failure and pulmonary oedema.

Treatment

- Empty the stomach and give activated charcoal (see Decontamination).
- Monitor heart rate, blood pressure and temperature.
- *Diazepam is best avoided.* Acepromazine or a barbiturate is recommended for tremors or convulsions.
- Ensure adequate hydration.
- Beta-blockers for prolonged or severe tachycardia.
- Symptomatic and supportive care.

Prognosis

Favourable.

Taxus species exposure in dogs

Alternative names

Taxus baccata (European yew), *Taxus cuspidata* (Japanese yew), *Taxus baccata* 'Fastigiata' (Irish yew)

Description/Source

A slow-growing, evergreen shrub or tree. The seed is enclosed in a fleshy aril ('berry') that is green when unripe and red when ripe.

Toxicology

Taxine A and taxine B are found in all parts of the plant except the fleshy aril. Taxine B is cardiotoxic and inhibits sodium and calcium currents. Also present are an irritant volatile oil, ephedrine and the cardiac glycoside taxiphyllin.

Risk factors

None known.

Clinical effects

Onset

Within 6 hours.

Taxus sp. ©Elizabeth Dauncey

Common signs

Vomiting, diarrhoea, hypersalivation, dilated pupils, lethargy, trembling and ataxia.

Other signs

Hypothermia, bradycardia, hypotension, respiratory depression, arrhythmias, convulsions and coma.

Treatment
- Empty the stomach and give activated charcoal (see Decontamination).
- Symptomatic and supportive care.

Prognosis
Favourable.

Toad venom exposure in dogs

For exposure in cats – see page 154

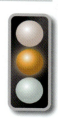

Description/Source
Two toads are native to Britain: the common toad (*Bufo bufo*); and the extremely rare natterjack toad (*Bufo calamita*). Most exposures occur during the summer months when toads are spawning.

Toxicology
All *Bufo* species of toads have parotid glands that secrete venom when the toad is threatened. All toads secrete similar venom; however, the toxicity of the venom varies between species. The venom contains various cardiotoxic substances, catecholamines and indole alkylamines. Serious poisonings are rare in Britain.

Risk factors
None known.

Clinical effects

Onset
Often within a few minutes; most effects occur within 30 to 60 minutes.

Common signs
Hypersalivation, frothing or foaming at the mouth, vomiting, erythematous mucous membranes, vocalizing, anxiety, ataxia and shaking.

Other signs
Twitching, tachycardia or bradycardia, hyperthermia, convulsions, coma and arrhythmias.

Treatment
- Gut decontamination is not required.
- Decontaminate the oral cavity by flushing with water.
- Monitor pulse, respiration and temperature.

- Atropine can be used for hypersalivation or bradycardia.
- Cooling measures may be required.
- Symptomatic and supportive care.

Prognosis

Excellent.

Tramadol exposure in dogs

For exposure in cats – see page 155

Description/Source

Tramadol is an opioid analgesic used to treat mild to moderate pain.

Toxicology

Tramadol has a low affinity for opiate receptors but may have some selectivity for the mu receptor. The main analgesic effect is thought to be inhibition of the reuptake of noradrenaline and serotonin.

Risk factors

None known.

Clinical effects

Onset

Usually within 2 hours, but may be delayed if a sustained release preparation has been ingested.

Common signs

Drowsiness, lethargy, depression, ataxia, vomiting and hypersalivation.

Other signs

Potentially, cyanosis, hypothermia, coma, and convulsions although severe toxicity in dogs after tramadol ingestion is very rare.

Treatment

- Empty the stomach and give activated charcoal (see Decontamination).
- Warming measures if required.
- Naloxone can be given for severe respiratory or central nervous system depression.
- Symptomatic and supportive care.

Prognosis

Favourable.

A B C D E F G H I J K L M N O P Q R S T U V W X Y Z

Tremorgenic mycotoxin exposure in dogs

Alternative name

Mycotoxin, penitrem A, roquefortine

Description/Source

Mycotoxins are fungal metabolites that cause toxicity in humans and animals. Tremorgenic mycotoxins are present in some mouldy foods (particularly dairy food such as cheese), in silage and compost, and can also occur in mouldy fallen fruit and nuts. There are a number of tremorgenic mycotoxins but only a few are of clinical significance. Penitrem A and roquefortine are most commonly associated with acute poisoning in small animals.

Toxicology

The mechanism of action is unclear and may vary with the mycotoxin. Penitrem A may interfere with the release of neurotransmitters.

Risk factors

None known.

Clinical effects

Onset

Usually within 30 minutes, but sometimes up to 3 hours.

Common signs

Vomiting, irritability, ataxia, muscle tremors, rigidity with hyperextension of extremities, hyperactivity, hyperaesthesia, tachycardia, panting, tachypnoea, nystagmus and dilated pupils. In severe cases, tremors, opisthotonus, convulsions and coma. Increased muscle activity can lead to hyperthermia, exhaustion, rhabdomyolysis, dehydration, hypoglycaemia, and raised lactate dehydrogenase, creatine kinase and liver enzymes.

Other signs

There is a risk of aspiration of vomit.

Treatment

- Empty the stomach and give repeat doses of activated charcoal (see Decontamination).
- Ensure adequate hydration and give antiemetics if required.

- Cooling measures may be required.
- Diazepam is ineffective in most cases and other drugs will be needed (e.g. pentobarbital, phenobarbital, propofol, methocarbamol).
- General anaesthesia may be required in unresponsive cases.
- Consider use of intravenous lipid emulsion in a severe case unresponsive to other therapies.
- Symptomatic and supportive care.

Prognosis

Favourable if mild signs occur. Poor if convulsions are uncontrolled.

Tricyclic antidepressant exposure in dogs

Alternative names

TCAs. Examples: amitriptyline, clomipramine, dosulepin (dothiepin), doxepin, imipramine, lofepramine, nortriptyline, trimipramine

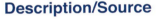

Description/Source

Used for behavioural disorders in dogs and as antidepressants in humans.

Toxicology

Tricyclic antidepressants are thought to act by blocking the re-uptake of noradrenaline and serotonin (5-HT) in the central nervous system. They also block the parasympathetic nervous system and the peripheral re-uptake of noradrenaline and have a membrane-stabilizing effect on the myocardium mediated by disruption of the sodium/potassium pump. Toxicity is possible at therapeutic doses, but more likely in overdose.

Risk factors

None known.

Clinical effects

Onset

Usually within 4 hours.

Common signs

Hyperexcitability, vomiting, ataxia and tremors are common. Dilated pupils, dry mucous membranes, urine retention, hypotension and tachycardia.

Other signs

Drowsiness or coma, respiratory depression, metabolic acidosis, hypokalaemia, convulsions, electrocardiogram changes (particularly prolonged QRS) and ventricular arrhythmias.

Treatment

- Empty the stomach and give activated charcoal (see Decontamination).
- Intravenous fluids for hypotension.
- If possible, monitor electrocardiogram and check electrolytes and blood gases.
- Diazepam for hyperexcitability or convulsions.
- Sodium bicarbonate is recommended for acidosis, tachycardia or electrocardiogram changes. Administration should be based on blood gas results; maintaining the blood pH above 7.5 can reverse TCA-induced cardiotoxicity.
- Symptomatic and supportive care.

Prognosis

Favourable.

Venlafaxine exposure in dogs

Description/Source

A serotonin noradrenaline reuptake inhibitor (SNRI) antidepressant used in humans.

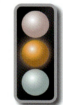

Toxicology

Venlafaxine acts by inhibition of neuronal uptake of noradrenaline, serotonin (5-HT) and, to a lesser extent, dopamine.

Risk factors

None known.

Clinical effects

Onset

Usually within 6 hours, but may be delayed if a sustained release preparation has been ingested.

Common signs

Dilated pupils, lethargy, drowsiness and ataxia.

Other signs

Vomiting, hyperthermia, vocalizing, hyperaesthesia, tachycardia and respiratory distress. Convulsions are rare. Arrhythmias have been reported in human overdose.

Treatment

- Empty the stomach and give activated charcoal (see Decontamination).
- Symptomatic and supportive care.

Prognosis

Favourable.

Viscum album exposure in dogs

Alternative name

European mistletoe (not to be confused with North American mistletoe, *Phoradendron serotinum*)

Description/Source

Mistletoe is a plant that lives on deciduous trees, sometimes as a parasite. The long stems have a woody appearance, and bear thick, dark green leaves. Clusters of yellowish flowers are produced in spring. The fruits are white, semi-translucent berries that contain a viscous juice and a single seed; they remain on the plant throughout winter. The plant is commonly available in the home as a Christmas decoration.

Toxicology

Although the berries, leaves and stems contain potentially toxic lectins and viscotoxins, this plant is considered to be of low acute toxicity.

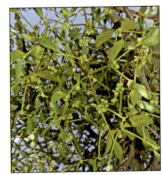

Viscum album.
©Elizabeth Dauncey

Risk factors

None known.

Clinical effects

Onset

Within a few hours.

Common signs

Vomiting, diarrhoea, hypersalivation and weakness.

Other signs

None.

Treatment

- Gut decontamination is not required, unless massive quantities have been consumed (see Decontamination).
- Ensure adequate hydration and give anti-emetics if required.
- Symptomatic and supportive care.

Prognosis

Excellent.

Vitamin D compound exposure in dogs

Description/Source

Vitamin D compounds such as calciferol (ergocalciferol, vitamin D2), colecalciferol (cholecalciferol, vitamin D3), calcipotriol, calcitriol, tacalcitol, alfacalcidol and paricalcitol are used in vitamin preparations, cod liver oil, veterinary medicines, growth promoters, rodenticides and human medicines (especially psoriasis creams).

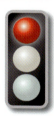

Toxicology

These compounds are rapidly absorbed and metabolized by the liver and kidney. Calcitriol is the major metabolite. Excess calcitriol results in hypercalcaemia, nephrotoxicity and tissue mineralization and calcification.

Risk factors

Pre-existing renal impairment.

Clinical effects

Onset

Usually 6 to 12 hours, but can be longer.

Common signs

Polydipsia, weakness, lethargy, profuse vomiting and diarrhoea, polyuria and signs of hypercalcaemia (anorexia, ataxia, arching of the back, muscle spasms, twitching and convulsions).

Other signs

Renal failure, cardiac function abnormalities, shock and pulmonary oedema.

Treatment

- Aggressive treatment is required.
- Empty the stomach and give activated charcoal (see Decontamination).
- Ensure adequate hydration and give anti-emetics if required.
- Monitor electrolyte concentrations and renal function.
- Gastroprotectants are recommended.
- Hypercalcaemia should be managed with isotonic (0.9%) sodium chloride infusion to promote diuresis plus furosemide and either bisphosphonates (e.g. pamidronate, clodronate) or calcitonin (4 to 7 IU/kg bodyweight s.c., q6-8h or every 2 to 3 hours, if needed). Hypercalcaemia may be severe and should be closely monitored.

Prognosis

Guarded if signs are severe or presentation is delayed. Poor if calcification of tissues has occurred.

Vitis vinifera fruits exposure in dogs

Alternative names

Grapevine fruits, grapes, currants, raisins, sultanas

Description/Source

The grapevine is cultivated for its fruit. In addition to use as grapes, they are also encountered as raisins, sultanas and currants and in products containing these, such as Christmas cake, Christmas pudding, fruit cake and chocolate raisins (see Chocolate).

Toxicology

The toxic mechanism is unknown and there appears to be no correlation between quantity ingested and clinical effects. Ingestion of the dried fruit, rather than grapes, is more likely to cause severe clinical effects.

Risk factors

None known.

Clinical effects

Onset

6 to 24 hours.

Common signs

Vomiting, diarrhoea, hypersalivation, haematemesis, bloody stools, anorexia, ataxia, weakness, lethargy and acute anuric renal failure.

Other signs

Haematuria, polydipsia and pancreatitis.

Treatment

- Empty the stomach and give repeat doses of activated charcoal (see Decontamination).
- Aggressive intravenous fluids to encourage diuresis with monitoring of renal function. If anuric renal failure develops, fluid therapy must be modified appropriately to avoid intravascular volume overload.
- Symptomatic and supportive care.

Prognosis

Favourable when treatment is started before onset of renal impairment. Guarded if signs of renal impairment are present.

Wallpaper adhesive exposure in dogs

Alternative name

Wallpaper paste

Description/Source

Adhesives used for sticking wall coverings to walls usually contain potato starch derivatives, polyvinyl acetate and fungicides to inhibit mould growth. They are available as powders to be mixed with water or as ready-to-use pastes.

Toxicology

Irritant to the gastrointestinal tract. The fungicides in these products are in a low concentration and of low acute toxicity.

Risk factors

None known.

Clinical effects

Onset
Within a few hours.

Common signs
Vomiting, diarrhoea, lethargy, inappetence and hypersalivation.

Other signs
Haematemesis, haemorrhagic diarrhoea, abdominal tenderness, tongue ulceration, weakness and hyperthermia.

Treatment
- Gut decontamination is not required.
- Ensure adequate hydration.
- Symptomatic and supportive care.

Prognosis
Excellent.

Xylitol exposure in dogs

Alternative name
Food additive E967

Description/Source
Xylitol is a sugar alcohol. It is used as a sweetener in confectionary and baking, and as an excipient in human and veterinary medications. It is also present in some drinking water additives for pets. Severe cases usually result from ingestion of chewing gums, sweets, and cakes baked with sugar substitute products.

Toxicology
A potent stimulator of insulin release in dogs. Xylitol exposures cause a dose-dependent rise in insulin concentrations, resulting in rapid-onset hypoglycaemia. Xylitol is also hepatotoxic.

Risk factors
None known.

Clinical effects

Onset
Hypoglycaemia within 1 hour but up to 12 for chewing gum; hepatic effects 2–72 hours.

Common signs

Signs related to hypoglycaemia (vomiting, tachycardia, ataxia, drowsiness, coma, convulsions and collapse).

Other signs

Liver failure and coagulopathy (can occur in the absence of hypoglycaemia).

Treatment

- Aggressive treatment is required.
- Empty the stomach and give activated charcoal (see Decontamination).
- Monitor blood glucose, and supplement as necessary.
- Monitor liver function; liver protectants can be given.

Prognosis

Favourable where hypoglycaemia is controlled without complications. Poor if liver failure is present.

Zinc exposure in dogs

Description/Source

Ingestion of zinc-containing coins, zinc or zinc-coated foreign bodies (e.g. nuts and bolts, galvanized wire) and chronic ingestion of topical zinc oxide medication.

Toxicology

Severe intravascular haemolysis is the most consistent clinical finding in acute zinc poisoning but the cause is unclear; it is not immune-mediated. It may be due to inhibition of erythrocyte enzymes, direct damage to the erythrocyte membrane, or increased susceptibility of erythrocyte to oxidative damage.

Risk factors

None known.

Clinical effects

Onset

Variable.

Common signs

Gastrointestinal signs, then haemolytic anaemia with haemoglobinuria, anorexia and depression.

Other signs
Convulsions, pancreatitis, disseminated intravascular haemolysis, renal and liver dysfunction.

Treatment
- Ensure adequate hydration and give anti-emetics if required.
- Radiography may confirm ingestion of a foreign body. Gut decontamination is unlikely to be effective for a foreign body and surgery or endoscopy for removal may be required.
- *Activated charcoal is not effective.*
- Famotidine or omeprazole may be given to reduce gastric acidity and reduce zinc absorption.
- Chelation is controversial; zinc concentrations should fall rapidly once the object has been removed.
- Monitor haematology.
- Blood transfusions may be required in severe cases.
- Symptomatic and supportive care.

Prognosis
Favourable in animals with mild to moderate signs. Guarded in animals with severe poisoning.

Zopiclone exposure in dogs

For exposure in cats – see page 157

Description/Source
A cyclopyrrolone hypnotic, used in the short-term treatment of insomnia in humans.

Toxicology
Zopiclone is unrelated to benzodiazepines. It acts on the neurotransmitter gamma-aminobutyric acid (GABA) receptor complex but at a different site to benzodiazepines. It has sedative, anticonvulsant and muscle relaxant effects. The individual response is variable and not dose-related.

Risk factors
None known.

Clinical effects

Onset
Usually within 4 hours.

Common signs

Drowsiness, ataxia, lethargy and vomiting.

Other signs

Paradoxically, in some dogs there may be hyperactivity, hyperaesthesia, hypersalivation, tachycardia, agitation, aggression and hyperthermia. Hypotension, coma and respiratory depression have been reported in human cases.

Treatment

- Empty the stomach and give activated charcoal (see Decontamination).
- Flumazenil could be considered in animals with severe respiratory or central nervous system depression but it is rarely required. *Dosage*: 0.01–0.02 mg/kg i.v., repeated after about 30 minutes, if required.
- Symptomatic and supportive care.

Prognosis

Favourable.

Alkali exposure in cats

Alternative names

Examples: sodium hydroxide (caustic soda, lye), potassium hydroxide (caustic potash), calcium hydroxide, sodium metasilicate

Description/Source

Present in a number of household products, particularly drain cleaners, oven cleaners, some paint strippers and some dishwasher products. Sodium hydroxide can be purchased as a household chemical for cleaning.

Toxicology

Alkalis cause liquefactive necrosis with saponification of fats and solubilization of proteins; they are also hygroscopic and will absorb water from the tissues. These effects result in adherence and deep penetration into tissue. The severity of injury will depend on the duration of contact, the volume ingested, and the concentration and pH of the substance involved. After ingestion, alkalis cause the most severe corrosive damage to the oesophagus, but the greater the volume ingested, the greater the risk of duodenal and gastric damage. Alkali burns of the eye are very serious because they cause disruption of the protective permeability barriers and rapidly penetrate the cornea and anterior chamber.

Risk factors

None known.

Clinical effects

Onset

Soon (may be within minutes) after exposure, but note that alkali burns may be painless initially, and may not be immediately evident. Onset of burns depends on concentration and volume of alkali, and duration of contact.

Common signs

- **After ingestion:** Burning pain in the mouth, oesophagus and stomach, with swelling of the lips, vomiting, haematemesis, hypersalivation, ulcerative mucosal burns, dyspnoea, stridor, dysphagia and shock. Oesophageal and pharyngeal oedema may occur.
- **Skin or eye contact:** Deep penetrating burns and necrosis.

Other signs

Acute complications include gastrointestinal haemorrhage and perforation, and upper airway obstruction. Oesophageal stricture can occur as a late complication.

Treatment

After ingestion:

- *Gut decontamination is contraindicated because of the risks of further injury on re-exposure of the oesophagus.*
- *Neutralizing chemicals should never be given because heat is produced during neutralization and this could exacerbate any injury.*
- Activated charcoal is of no benefit.
- Oral fluids may be given unless there is evidence of severe injury.
- Endoscopy may be required to assess severity of injury.
- Gastroprotectants (antacids, H2 blockers, sucralfate) can be given but will have limited effectiveness in the face of ulceration.
- Analgesia will be required. If gastric ulceration is present NSAIDs should be avoided.
- Steroids can be given but not if there is evidence of gastric ulceration. They may be more useful in the healing phase to prevent fibrosis.
- Symptomatic and supportive care.

Skin or eye contact:

- Prolonged copious irrigation with water or saline is required to decontaminate skin and eyes effectively (see Decontamination).
- If possible, the pH of the skin/eye should be tested 15 minutes after decontamination and irrigation repeated if the affected area is still alkaline.
- Symptomatic and supportive care.

Prognosis

Guarded, depending on the severity of injury.

Alphachloralose exposure in cats

For exposure in dogs – see page 6

Alternative name

Chloralose

Description/Source

A rodenticide for mice and rats; also used to control pest birds. Baits are available in various forms, including wheat or bran granules containing 2 to 4%. Professional products may be more concentrated.

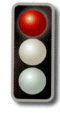

Toxicology

Alphachloralose possesses both stimulant and depressant properties. At low exposures it causes excitation by suppressing the descending inhibitory mechanisms in the nervous system. At higher doses it acts as a central nervous system depressant through neuronal suppression in the ascending reticular activating system.

Risk factors

None known.

Clinical effects

Onset

Usually within 1–2 hours.

Common signs

Initially ataxia, aggression and hyperaesthesia. Then drowsiness, weakness, twitching, tremor, constricted or dilated pupils, hypothermia, coma and convulsions.

Other signs

Respiratory failure and hyperthermia (from repeated convulsions).

Treatment

- Empty the stomach (see Decontamination).
- Activated charcoal is not useful.
- Monitor respiration and temperature.
- Diazepam can be used for tremors, twitching or convulsions but other drugs may be required (e.g. pentobarbital, phenobarbital).
- Warming measures if patient is hypothermic and cooling measures if patient is hyperthermic.
- Symptomatic and supportive care.

Prognosis

Favourable with prompt treatment.

Benzalkonium chloride (BAC) exposure in cats

Description/Source

Quaternary ammonium compound (QAC), which is classified as a cationic detergent and used as a domestic and industrial disinfectant. Also found in some patio cleaners.

Toxicology

The main effects of benzalkonium chloride are due to its irritancy, which results in local tissue damage. Cats are often presented hours or days after exposure.

Risk factors

None known.

Clinical effects

Onset

Can be up to 12 hours.

Common signs

Hypersalivation, vomiting, inappetence, diarrhoea and ulceration of the tongue and oral mucosa. On the skin there may be erythema, inflammation, ulceration and hair loss.

Other signs

Dehydration, depression, hyperthermia and respiratory effects.

Treatment

- *Gut decontamination is not recommended.*
- If dermal exposure was recent, decontaminate by rinsing thoroughly with water (see Decontamination).
- Analgesia will probably be required.
- Ensure adequate hydration.
- In the case of severe oral irritation, nutritional support may be required through the use of feeding tubes.
- Symptomatic and supportive care.

Prognosis

Favourable.

Benzodiazepine exposure in cats

For exposure in dogs – see page 18

Alternative names

Examples: alprazolam, bromazepam, chlordiazepoxide, clobazam, clonazepam, clorazepate, diazepam, flunitrazepam, flurazepam, loprazolam, lorazepam, lormetazepam, midazolam, nitrazepam, oxazepam, temazepam

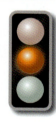

Description/Source

Benzodiazepines are used as sedatives, anxiolytics, anticonvulsants and premedicants.

Toxicology

Benzodiazepines enhance the effect of the inhibitory neurotransmitter gamma-aminobutyric acid (GABA).

Risk factors

None known.

Clinical effects

Onset

Usually within 2 hours. Idiosyncratic hepatic necrosis can occur within 4 days of initiation of diazepam administration.

Common signs

Ataxia, incoordination and drowsiness.

Other signs

Tremor, lethargy, depression, weakness, vomiting, hypothermia, nystagmus, disorientation, polydipsia and polyphagia, coma, hypotension and respiratory depression. Some animals develop paradoxical stimulation, with hyperactivity, hyperaesthesia, agitation, restlessness, aggression and hyperthermia. Idiosyncratic hepatic necrosis can occur in cats on diazepam therapy.

Treatment

- Give activated charcoal (see Decontamination).
- Symptomatic and supportive care.
- Flumazenil could be considered in animals with severe respiratory or central nervous system depression. *Dosage*: 0.01–0.02 mg/kg i.v., repeated after about 30 minutes, if required.

Prognosis

Favourable.

Carbamate insecticide exposure in cats

For exposure in dogs – see page 27

Alternative names

Examples: aldicarb, bendiocarb, carbaryl, carbofuran, fenoxycarb, methiocarb, methomyl, oxamyl, thiodicarb

Description/Source

Carbamate insecticides are widely used as garden and household pesticides, and in agriculture. Formulations include liquids, sprays and powders which may be used as supplied or diluted. Domestic products usually contain a low concentration; agricultural products are more hazardous.

Toxicology

Carbamates act in a similar way to organophosphates, binding to and inhibiting acetylcholinesterase. This results in accumulation of the neurotransmitter acetylcholine and activation of nicotinic and muscarinic receptors. Therefore both nicotinic and muscarinic effects occur, although nicotinic receptors rapidly become desensitized. Effects resulting from carbamate poisoning tend to be of much shorter duration compared with those of organophosphate poisoning and use of cholinesterase reactivators (such as pralidoxime) is unnecessary.

Risk factors

None known.

Clinical effects

Onset

Usually within 15 minutes to 3 hours.

Common signs

Mild to moderate effects normally include hypersalivation, increased bronchial secretion, ataxia, diarrhoea, constricted pupils, muscle fasciculation, tremors and twitching, weakness, shaking, hyperaesthesia, pyrexia, restlessness and urinary incontinence.

Other signs

Collapse, bradycardia, respiratory depression, convulsions, cyanosis and coma may occur in severe cases. Myopathy occurs rarely following recovery.

Treatment

- Empty the stomach and give activated charcoal (see Decontamination).
- Decontaminate the skin by washing with a mild detergent and lukewarm water (see Decontamination).
- Body temperature should be maintained, and blood gases and electrolytes monitored and corrected.
- Symptomatic and supportive care.
- Atropine should be given to reverse cholinergic effects.

Prognosis

Favourable with aggressive supportive care.

Chlorophytum comosum exposure in cats

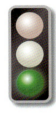

Alternative names
Spider plant, ribbon plant

Description/Source
A very common houseplant with long thin variegated leaves with longitudinal stripes of white, cream or pale green, arranged in a rosette.

Toxicology
This plant contains saponins, which have a bitter, acrid taste and local irritant effects on mucous membranes. However, it is considered to be of low toxicity.

Risk factors
None known.

Clinical effects

Onset
Within a few hours of ingestion.

Common signs
Hypersalivation, vomiting, inappetence and lethargy.

Other signs
Dehydration and depression.

Treatment
- Gut decontamination is not required.
- Symptomatic and supportive care.

Prognosis
Excellent.

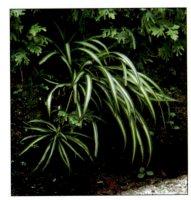

Chlorophytum sp.
Courtesy of Matti Nissalo and
Lahiru Wijedasa

Cordyline and *Dracaena* species exposure in cats

Description/Source

These plants are closely related.

- *Cordyline* species are evergreen trees and shrubs grown as foliage plants. They usually have a single stem and several branches that are topped with a crown of leaves.
- *Dracaena* species are common foliage houseplants; there are many varieties. Leaves may be: narrow, leathery or stiff; striped pink and yellow; or red-edged or deep glossy green. *Dracaena draco* (dragon tree), *Dracaena marginata* (Madagascan dragon tree), *Dracaena sanderiana* (ribbon dracaena, marketed as lucky bamboo).

Toxicology

The toxic mechanism is unknown, but the plants contain cytotoxic saponins.

Risk factors

None known.

Clinical effects

Onset

Usually within a few hours.

Common signs

Hypersalivation, vomiting, inappetence, lethargy and ataxia.

Other signs

Dilated pupils, pyrexia, abdominal discomfort, dehydration, leucocytosis and limb oedema.

Treatment

- Gut decontamination is unlikely to be required.
- IV fluids for rehydration and antiemetics for persistent vomiting.

Prognosis

Favourable.

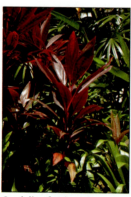

Cordyline fruticosa.
Courtesy of Matti Nissalo and Lahiru Wijedasa

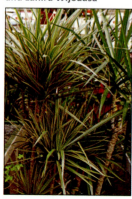

Dracaena sp.
©Elizabeth Dauncey

Cyclamen species exposure in cats

Description/Source

Flowering, herbaceous plants found in woods, hedgerows and grassy places, and grown as ornamental garden and houseplants. The leaves and flowers sprout in rosettes from a flattened tuber. The leaf shape and colour are variable depending on the species. In most species, leaves from the previous autumn wither and die in summer. Flowering may occur at any time of year, depending on the species. The stem is bent at the tip, so that the white, pink or purple flower faces downwards.

Toxicology

The plant contains triterpenoid saponins, which have an acrid, rancid taste, so ingestion of a significant quantity is unlikely. Saponins have local irritant effects on mucous membranes, as well as systemic effects, but the exact mechanism of action is unknown. They are not well absorbed from the gastrointestinal tract and severe clinical effects from acute exposures are therefore unlikely.

Risk factors

None known.

Clinical effects

Onset

4 to 6 hours.

Common signs

Hypersalivation, inappetence, vomiting and diarrhoea.

Other signs

Allergic reactions may occur.

Treatment

- Gut decontamination is unlikely to be required.
- Allow access to oral fluids.
- Symptomatic and supportive care.

Prognosis

Favourable.

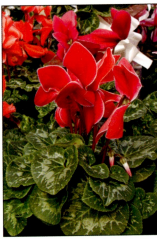

Cyclamen sp.
©Elizabeth Dauncey

Dichlorophen exposure in cats

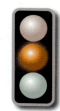

Description/Source

Anthelmintic used for the treatment of tapeworm infection in cats and dogs.

Toxicology

The mechanism of toxicity is thought to involve the uncoupling of oxidative phosphorylation. Some animals may exhibit signs at a therapeutic dose.

Risk factors

None known

Clinical effects

Onset

Usually within 3 hours, sometimes up to 12 hours.

Common signs

Vomiting, hypersalivation, ataxia, lethargy, anorexia, tachycardia, pyrexia, hyperaesthesia and collapse.

Other signs

Inappetence, hyperventilation, dilated pupils, dyspnoea and disorientation.

Treatment

- Empty the stomach (see Decontamination).
- Give activated charcoal in acute cases (see Decontamination).
- Symptomatic and supportive care.

Prognosis

Excellent.

Essential oil exposure in cats

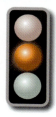

Alternative names

Examples: clove oil, eucalyptus oil, peppermint oil, pine oil, tea tree (*Melaleuca*) oil

Description/Source

Oils of botanical origin. They have many applications, being used in shampoos, insect and animal repellents, air fresheners and room deodorizers. Tea tree (*Melaleuca*) oil is commonly implicated in feline poisoning. Poisonings occur as a result of inappropriate dermal application of products to cats. Cats rarely drink the oil itself but can ingest it while grooming themselves or housemates.

Toxicology

Essential oils are generally highly lipophilic and thus rapidly absorbed from the gastrointestinal tract if ingested. They are irritant to mucous membranes and many may have significant systemic effects. They are also volatile and there is a significant risk of aspiration upon vomiting, retching or coughing.

Risk factors

None known.

Clinical effects

Onset

Usually within 2 hours.

Common signs

Systemic signs can occur from dermal or oral exposure. Signs are variable, depending on the oil and concentration. Hypersalivation, depression, lethargy, ataxia, tremor and abdominal discomfort are common after ingestion. Alopecia and skin burns may occur after dermal exposure.

Other signs

Weakness, collapse, coma and convulsions. The breath, vomitus, urine and faeces may smell of the oil. Elevated liver enzymes and renal impairment may occur. If aspirated, abnormal lung sounds, wheezing, coughing, dyspnoea and respiratory distress consistent with pneumonitis.

Treatment

Ingestion:
- Rinse mouth areas cautiously with water.
- *Do not induce vomiting,* owing to volatility and potential pulmonary risks.
- Ensure adequate hydration.
- Respiratory effects should be managed conventionally.
- Symptomatic and supportive care.
- In the case of severe oral irritation, nutritional support may be required through the use of feeding tubes.

Skin contact:
- Wash thoroughly with simple soaps or detergents and water, ensuring that rinsing is very thorough. Be careful to avoid hypothermia

- It is advisable to place an Elizabethan collar on the animal to prevent further grooming.

Prognosis

Favourable in animals with mild to moderate effects. Guarded in animals with respiratory or severe neurological signs.

Ethylene glycol exposure in cats

For exposure in dogs – see page 42

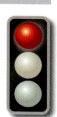

Alternative name

Ethanediol

Description/Source

Used widely as an antifreeze (often dyed a bright colour), in screen washes, brake fluid, inks, and as a coolant.

Toxicology

Ethylene glycol is converted by alcohol dehydrogenase to a number of toxic metabolites, and it is these compounds that are responsible for the renal damage and hypocalcaemia. Ethylene glycol has a lower fatal dose and higher mortality rate in cats than in dogs.

Risk factors

None known.

Clinical effects

Onset

Initial signs from 30 minutes to 12 hours. In cats, the onset of effects may be more rapid than in dogs.

Common signs

- **Stage 1 (30 minutes to 12 hours):** Central nervous system signs with vomiting, ataxia, weakness and convulsions. Metabolic acidosis (high anion gap) and hypocalcaemia.
- **Stages 2 and 3 (12 to 24 hours):** Cardiopulmonary signs with tachycardia, tachypnoea and pulmonary oedema. There may be a transient recovery followed by coma and convulsions. Renal signs with oliguria, azotaemia and renal failure.

Other signs

Oxaluria, hyperglycaemia, hyperkalaemia and hyperphosphataemia.

Treatment

- Gut decontamination is probably only worthwhile if the animal presents within 1 hour of ingestion (see Decontamination).
- Activated charcoal is not useful.
- Ethanol is a specific antidote and should be given as soon as possible. **Ethanol should not be given to cats in renal failure.**
- Sodium bicarbonate can be used for acidosis.
- Monitor renal function.
- Supportive care.

Prognosis

Guarded for animals that present early. Poor in animals with renal failure.

Euphorbia pulcherrima exposure in cats

Alternative name

Poinsettia

Description/Source

An ornamental perennial houseplant commonly available as a pot plant at Christmas. It grows up to 25–40 cm high and has large green leaves. The flowers are very small and surrounded by large red (sometimes white, cream, pink or multicoloured) bracts, which are often mistaken for petals.

Toxicology

Poinsettia has the reputation of being a toxic plant but this is generally not the case. *Euphorbia* species contain diterpene esters but concentrations in poinsettia are very low compared to other species. Irritant effects are typically observed after ingestion. Severe cases of poisoning are rarely reported in pets.

Risk factors

None known.

Clinical effects

Onset

Effects are usually rapid in onset and self-limiting.

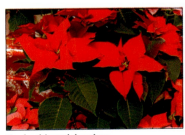

Euphorbia pulcherrima.
©Elizabeth Dauncey

Common signs
Vomiting, hypersalivation, anorexia, lethargy and depression.

Other signs
None.

Treatment
- Gut decontamination is not required.
- Ensure adequate hydration.
- Symptomatic and supportive care.

Prognosis
Excellent.

Fabric washing product exposure in cats

Description/Source
Liquid, powder or gels, detergents and fabric conditioners used in hand- or machine-washing of fabrics. Many contain some enzymatic components, as well as buffers and preservatives.

Toxicology
Most of the chemicals used in fabric cleaning products are irritants only, although products are increasingly presented in compact and therefore concentrated forms.

Risk factors
None known.

Clinical effects

Onset
Within 4 hours.

Common signs
Vomiting, hypersalivation, retching, diarrhoea and gastrointestinal discomfort. Grooming of contaminated fur or ingestion of concentrated solutions may cause severe buccal and lingual irritation, inappetence and dehydration. Dermal exposures can result in erythema, dermatitis and, rarely, skin burns.

Other signs

Aspiration of detergents upon vomiting or retching could result in aspiration pneumonitis.

Treatment

- Gut decontamination is not recommended.
- If appropriate, clean the skin (see Decontamination).
- Consider isolating the animal and placing an Elizabethan collar.
- Ensure adequate hydration.
- If evidence of respiratory signs, check lung sounds and obtain chest X-ray if required.
- Symptomatic and supportive care.
- Nutritional support may be required if oral ulceration is severe.

Prognosis

Favourable in animals with mild to moderate effects. Guarded in animals with severe respiratory signs.

Fluoroquinolone antibiotic exposure in cats

Alternative names

Examples: danofloxacin, difloxacin, enrofloxacin, ibafloxacin, marbofloxacin

Description/Source

Antibiotics active against a wide range of Gram-negative bacteria.

Toxicology

These drugs inhibit bacterial DNA gyrase (a type II topoisomerase), thereby preventing replication and synthesis of bacterial DNA. They are well tolerated. However, exposure to a large quantity can cause convulsions because these drugs can act as gamma-aminobutyric acid (GABA) antagonists and bind to the N-methyl-D-aspartate (NMDA) receptor.

Risk factors

Old age, renal or hepatic impairment (for retinal degeneration, a rare and idiosyncratic reaction seen particularly with enrofloxacin).

Clinical effects

Onset

Usually within a few hours.

Common signs

Gastrointestinal signs with vomiting, hypersalivation, inappetence, soft faeces or diarrhoea, anorexia and lethargy.

Other signs

Ataxia, tremor and convulsions can occur following very large overdose. Risk of blindness from high doses or high plasma concentration.

Treatment

- Gut decontamination is probably only required after a large acute ingestion. Empty the stomach and give activated charcoal (see Decontamination).
- Ensure adequate hydration.
- Diazepam for convulsions.
- Symptomatic and supportive care.

Prognosis

Favourable.

Glyphosate exposure in cats

For exposure in dogs – see page 51

Description/Source

Glyphosate is a broad-spectrum post-emergence herbicide; it is an organophosphate herbicide with no anticholinesterase activity.

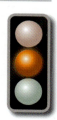

Toxicology

The irritant surfactant polyoxyethylene amine (POEA), which is present in many liquid preparations, may be responsible for some of the effects reported. Some products contain up to 15% surfactant. The toxic mechanisms of glyphosate are unknown, but may be related to uncoupling of oxidative phosphorylation. Ingestion of treated plant material is likely to result in only mild gastrointestinal effects.

Risk factors

None known.

Clinical effects

Onset

30 minutes to 6 hours.

Common signs

Gastric irritation (hypersalivation, abdominal pain, vomiting and diarrhoea), lethargy, hyper- or hypothermia, polydipsia, ataxia and weakness. Respiratory complications (cyanosis, tachypnoea, dyspnoea, pulmonary oedema, bronchopneumonia) are common. Eye and skin irritation may occur.

Other signs

Collapse, dilated pupils, hyperaesthesia, twitching, tremor, convulsions, bradycardia, elevated liver enzymes and renal failure.

Treatment

- Give activated charcoal (see Decontamination).
- Gut decontamination by emesis or gastric lavage is best avoided because of the risk of respiratory complications in cats.
- Check lung sounds in all symptomatic cats.
- Ensure adequate hydration and give anti-emetics if required.
- Check renal and liver function.
- Symptomatic and supportive care.

Prognosis

Favourable in most cases. Guarded in animals with respiratory complications.

Imidacloprid ingestion in cats

Description/Source

Ectoparasiticide (a chloronicotinyl nitroguanide insecticide) for the control of fleas in cats, dogs and rabbits; available as a topical spot-on pipette. Also used as an agrochemical. Most cases of toxicity in cats are due to ingestion while grooming themselves or another cat.

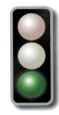

Toxicology

Imidacloprid binds to the acetylcholine receptor on the post-synaptic portion of insect nerve cells and prevents binding of acetylcholine. This stops the transmission of nerve impulses, resulting in paralysis and death of the insect. Imidacloprid is of low toxicity in mammals because of the lower concentration of nicotinic acetylcholine receptors in mammalian nervous tissue compared to insects.

Risk factors

None known.

Clinical effects

Onset

Immediate.

Common signs

Hypersalivation, vomiting and anorexia.

Other signs

Ataxia, hyperaesthesia, twitching and tremor. Inflammation, tongue ulceration and dysphagia can occur after accidental oral administration.

Treatment

- Gut decontamination is not required.
- Oral fluids may be given.
- Symptomatic and supportive care.

Prognosis

Excellent.

Lilium and *Hemerocallis* species exposure in cats

Alternative name

Lilies

Description/Source

Common house or garden plants with showy flowers, grown from bulbs. May also be present in bouquets of flowers. **Note:** The *Lilium* species are the true lilies: *Lilium asiatica* (Asiatic lily); *Lilium hydridum* (Japanese showy lilies); *Lilium lancifolium* (synonym *Lilium tigrinium*) (tiger lily); *Lilium longiflorum* (Easter lily); *Lilium orientalis* (stargazer lily, oriental lily); *Lilium rubrum* (rubrum lily); *Lilium speciosum*; *Lilium umbellatum* (Western or wood lily). The day lily is *Hemerocallis* sp. Many other unrelated plants have lily in their common name.

Toxicology

All parts of the plant are nephrotoxic and cause necrosis of renal tubular epithelial cells. Mortality is high if treatment is not initiated within 18 to 24 hours of ingestion. The cause of the renal toxicity is unknown.

Risk factors

Pre-existing renal impairment.

Clinical effects

Onset

Usually 2 to 6 hours; biochemical changes of renal impairment from 18 to 24 hours.

Common signs

Vomiting, anorexia, depression and renal failure.

Other signs

Polyuria, polydipsia, pancreatitis and convulsions.

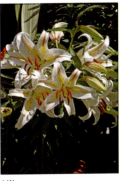

Lilium sp.
©Elizabeth Dauncey

Treatment

- Empty the stomach and give activated charcoal (see Decontamination).
- If there is pollen on the skin and fur, wash thoroughly (see Decontamination).
- Aggressive intravenous fluids and monitoring of renal function.
- Symptomatic and supportive care.

Prognosis

Favourable when treatment is started before onset of renal impairment. Guarded if signs of renal impairment are present.

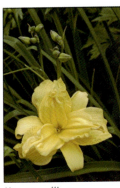

Hemerocallis sp.
©Elizabeth Dauncey

Luminous novelty exposure in cats

Description/Source

Novelty items such as glow-in-the-dark necklaces, glow sticks, fluorescent necklaces, bracelets and wands, are frequently available at Hallowe'en and Bonfire Night. They consist of plastic tubing filled with a liquid mixture that gives off light of various colours.

Toxicology

These products typically contain dibutyl phthalate, which is of low toxicity. The quantity ingested is usually small due to the unpleasant taste and systemic effects do not occur. Effects are usually mild and transient.

Risk factors

None known.

Clinical effects

Onset

Immediate.

Common signs

Hypersalivation.

Other signs

Frothing or foaming at the mouth, vomiting, aggression and hyperactivity.

Treatment

Oral fluids to remove the taste.

Prognosis

Excellent.

Metaldehyde exposure in cats

For exposure in dogs – see page 66

Description/Source

Metaldehyde is present in many molluscicide preparations. It is also found in fuel packs for camping stoves.

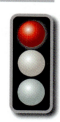

Toxicology

The mechanism of toxicity is not fully elucidated. It is suggested that toxicity results primarily from a decrease in inhibitory gamma-aminobutyric acid (GABA) concentrations.

Risk factors

None known.

Clinical effects

Onset

Extremely rapid, often within 30 minutes.

Common signs

Hyperaesthesia, tremors, twitching, convulsions, hyperthermia, panting, respiratory distress and cyanosis.

Other signs

Nystagmus, tachycardia and tachypnoea or respiratory depression.

Treatment

- Owing to rapid onset of severe clinical signs induction of emesis is potentially hazardous, but in potentially severe cases gastric lavage under anaesthesia should be considered (see Decontamination).
- Twitching or convulsions need aggressive management, initially with diazepam but with escalation to full anaesthesia using propofol or isoflurane.
- Cooling measures may be required.
- Symptomatic and supportive care.

Prognosis

Favourable if mild signs occur. Poor if convulsions are uncontrolled.

Milbemycin exposure in cats

For exposure in dogs – see page 70

Description/Source

Milbemycin is a macrocyclic lactone anthelmintic, used alone or with other anthelmintics.

Toxicology

Milbemycin increases nematode and insect membrane permeability to chloride ions via glutamate-gated chloride ion channels. This leads to hyperpolarization of the neuromuscular membrane and flaccid paralysis and death of the parasite. Neurological signs can occur in cats.

Risk factors

Young age.

Clinical effects

Onset

Generally 2–12 hours..

Common signs

Ataxia, tremor, twitching and collapse.

Other signs

Hyperaesthesia, drowsiness, hypothermia and coma.

Treatment

- Empty the stomach and give activated charcoal (see Decontamination).
- Consider use of intravenous lipid emulsion in a severe case unresponsive to other therapies.
- Symptomatic and supportive care.

Prognosis

Favourable in most cases but guarded in cats with significant neurological signs.

Neem oil exposure in cats

Alternative names

Margosa oil, margosa extract

Description/Source

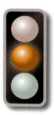

A bitter and inedible oil from the seed of the Asian tree *Azadirachta indica*. It is widely used in herbal medicine and contains numerous compounds including the insecticide azadirachtin. It is used as a flea treatment for cats.

Toxicology

The toxic mechanism is unknown.

Risk factors

None known.

Clinical effects

Onset

30 minutes to 48 hours.

Common signs

Lethargy, disorientation, hypersalivation, anorexia, abdominal discomfort, vomiting, diarrhoea, ataxia, tachycardia, tremor, twitching, muscle fasciculations, hyperaesthesia, convulsions and hyperthermia.

Other signs

Renal failure and elevation of liver enzymes. Local irritation, ulceration and hair loss may occur at the site of application.

Treatment

- If the cat is showing serious clinical signs, decontaminate by washing with a mild detergent and lukewarm water (see Decontamination).
- Symptomatic and supportive care.
- Check liver and renal function.

Prognosis

Favourable if no neurological effects occur. Guarded if convulsions occur.

Nepeta cataria exposure in cats

Alternative names

Catnip, catmint, catrup

Description/Source

A hardy upright perennial herb with white-purple flowers from July to September. It has a strong mint-like odour and taste. It is commonly available in toys and treats for cats. Cats find the plant attractive and respond to nepetalactone in the fresh or dried plant, juice or extract. Not all cats respond to catnip; it is thought to be an autosomal dominant trait.

Toxicology

Catnip contains *cis-trans*-nepetalactone, valeric acid and an essential oil containing *cis-trans*-nepetalactone and nepetalic acid.

Risk factors

None known.

Clinical effects

Onset

Within a few minutes.

Common signs

Catnip is not harmful to cats. They sniff, lick and chew the

Nepeta cataria.
© Bruce Works | Dreamstime.com

leaves (or toy) with head shaking, and chin and cheek rubbing. There may be hypersalivation, apparent hallucinations, sexual stimulation or vocalization.

Other signs

The signs reported are probably due to euphoria.

Treatment

None required.

Prognosis

Excellent.

Nitenpyram exposure in cats

For exposure in dogs – see page 74

Description/Source

Nitenpyram is a neonicotinoid insecticide used orally in cats and dogs for the control of fleas.

Toxicology

Nitenpyram inhibits nicotinic acetylcholine receptors in insects but does not inhibit acetylcholinesterase. It is considered to be of low toxicity in mammals. Doses of up to 10 times the therapeutic level have been well tolerated in cats.

Risk factors

None known.

Clinical effects

Onset

1 to 2 hours.

Common signs

Increased scratching, hypersalivation, hyperaesthesia, vomiting and diarrhoea. Hyperactivity and panting.

Other signs

Tachypnoea and tachycardia.

Treatment

- Gut decontamination is not required as severe effects are not expected.
- Symptomatic and supportive care.

Prognosis

Favourable.

Nitroscanate exposure in cats

For exposure in dogs – see page 75

Description/Source

Nitroscanate is an isothiocyanate anthelmintic used in dogs. It is not approved for use in cats.

Toxicology

Nitroscanate is generally well tolerated in cats, even up to doses of 200 mg/kg. Effects do not appear to be dose-related and can occur with therapeutic doses or after a small overdose.

Risk factors

None known.

Clinical effects

Onset

1 to 12 hours.

Common signs

Ataxia and incoordination are the most common signs.

Other signs

Depression and inappentence.

Treatment

- Gut decontamination is probably not required unless a large dose has been ingested (see Decontamination).
- Symptomatic and supportive care.

Prognosis

Favourable.

Non-steroidal anti-inflammatory drug (NSAID) exposure in cats

For exposure in dogs – see page 76

Alternative names

Examples: aceclofenac, acemetacin, carprofen, celecoxib, dexibuprofen, dexketoprofen, diclofenac, etodolac, etoricoxib, fenbufen, flurbiprofen, ibuprofen, indometacin, ketoprofen, ketorolac, mavacoxib, meloxicam, nabumetone, naproxen, parecoxib, piroxicam, robenacoxib, sulindac, tiaprofenic acid, tolfenamic acid. See also Paracetamol.

Description/Source

NSAIDs have both analgesic and anti-inflammatory effects, and are used in the treatment of pain associated with inflammation. NSAIDs reduce the production of prostaglandins by inhibition of cyclooxygenase (COX) enzymes. Prostaglandins are involved in control of gastric acid production, stimulation of secretion of mucous and bicarbonate by the gastric epithelium and maintenance of mucosal blood flow. In the kidneys, prostaglandins take part in renal homeostasis. COX-1 is involved in the synthesis of regulatory prostaglandins, whereas COX-2 is inducible and is principally concerned with the synthesis of prostaglandins involved in the inflammatory response.

Toxicology

The toxicity of a particular NSAID depends on which isoform(s) of COX it inhibits, and to what extent. There is limited information on the toxicity of ibuprofen in cats. Many papers report that cats are twice as sensitive as dogs to ibuprofen due to their limited glucuronyl-conjugating ability but this is not supported by clinical evidence. In addition, oxidation is the main metabolic pathway in other animals and humans (although glucuronidation of some metabolites does occur).

Risk factors

Dehydration, hypotension, pre-existing renal insufficiency.

Clinical effects

Onset

Usually within 2 to 6 hours.

Common signs

Inappetence, vomiting, lethargy, diarrhoea, melaena, haematemesis, abdominal tenderness, ataxia, polydipsia and polyuria.

Other signs

Tremor, drowsiness, weakness, depression, gastrointestinal ulceration, convulsions and renal failure. Rarely, liver damage.

Treatment

- Empty the stomach and give activated charcoal (see Decontamination).
- Ensure adequate hydration and give anti-emetics if required.
- Check renal and liver function.
- Gastric protectants are recommended (see BSAVA Formulary).
- Use of prostaglandin analogue (misoprostol) is recommended.
- Symptomatic and supportive care.

Prognosis

Favourable if treated early. Guarded in animals with renal impairment.

Organophosphate insecticide exposure in cats

For exposure in dogs – see page 78

Alternative names

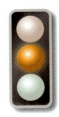

Examples: chlorfenvinphos, chlorpyrifos, demeton-*S*-methyl, dimpylate (diazinon), dichlorvos, dimethoate, fenitrothion, fenthion, heptenophos, malathion, pirimiphos-methyl

Description/Source

Garden, household and agricultural insecticides. **Note:** Some formulations contain petroleum distillate solvents.

Toxicology

Organophosphates (OPs) bind to and inhibit acetylcholinesterase, resulting in accumulation of the neurotransmitter acetylcholine and activation of nicotinic receptors. This results in both nicotinic and muscarinic effects, although nicotinic receptors rapidly become desensitized. OP insecticides are usually only present in low concentrations in domestic products and severe poisoning is uncommon. Agricultural products are more hazardous.

Risk factors

None known.

Clinical effects

Onset

Usually within 12 to 24 hours.

Common signs

Hypersalivation, ataxia, diarrhoea, constricted pupils, muscle fasciculation, tremors and twitching, weakness, shaking, hyperaesthesia, hyperthermia, restlessness and urinary incontinence.

Other signs

Bradycardia, respiratory depression, convulsions and coma. Some OP insecticides can cause delayed neuropathy.

Treatment

- Depending on the formulation, empty the stomach and give activated charcoal (see Decontamination).
- Decontaminate the skin by washing with a mild detergent and lukewarm water (see Decontamination).
- Atropine should be given to reverse cholinergic effects. Atropine acts as a non-competitive antagonist by blocking the effect of the muscarinic receptors on target organs.
- Cooling measures if required.
- Pralidoxime may be given in severe cases. Pralidoxime is a cholinesterase reactivator, which dephosphorylates acetylcholinesterase. It is most effective when used as an adjunct to atropine therapy.
- Symptomatic and supportive care.

Prognosis

Favourable.

Paint exposure in cats

Description/Source

Decorating and artist materials. Some paints are also designed to prevent climbing and fouling.

Toxicology

Emulsion, watercolour and acrylic paints are irritant to skin and mucous membranes only. Gloss paints, oil paints, solvent-based and anti-climb paints, generally being spirit-based, are also irritant but are harder to remove from contaminated fur. Ingestion may occur through grooming. Their solvent base means that aspiration- or inhalation-induced pneumonitis is a potential risk upon vomiting or if animals are confined in areas where paints have spilt. Ingestion of dried paint is not hazardous (unless the paint is old and contains lead).

Risk factors

None known.

Clinical effects

Onset

Within 4 hours.

Common signs

After ingestion: Retching, vomiting and hypersalivation. Gloss, oil, solvent and speciality paints may cause severe buccal and lingual irritation, inappetence and dehydration.

Contact with skin: Gloss, oil, solvent and speciality paints may cause significant irritation, drying and erythema of exposed skin.

Other signs

After ingestion: Aspiration of solvents upon vomiting or retching could result in aspiration pneumonitis.

Treatment

- For water-based paints decontaminate the skin by washing with a mild detergent and lukewarm water (see Decontamination).
- For all other paints the use of gel degreasants may be considered, although these will then need careful washing off. If unavailable, vegetable or baby oil can be used; these will also need to be thoroughly removed after decontamination.
- **Do not use white spirit, turpentine or turpentine substitute, or solvents to remove paint from skin.** Clip or shave fur if appropriate. Isolate and place an Elizabethan collar to prevent grooming.
- Ensure adequate hydration and nutrition.
- Assess respiratory function if appropriate.
- Symptomatic and supportive care.

Prognosis

Favourable.

Paracetamol exposure in cats

For exposure in dogs – see page 79

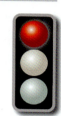

Alternative name

Acetaminophen

Description/Source

A non-narcotic analgesic with antipyretic properties, commonly found in combined oral analgesic preparations.

Toxicology

Paracetamol is metabolized in the liver by glucuronidation, sulphation and oxidation; the glucuronide and sulphate conjugates are non-toxic. Cats have a restricted ability to conjugate the drug with glucuronic acid, and thus sulphation becomes the primary route of excretion. However, this pathway becomes saturated at high doses, resulting in more oxidation. This results in a highly reactive metabolite that depletes glutathione stores and then binds with cellular macromolecules to bring about cellular necrosis. In addition, metabolites induce methaemoglobin and Heinz body formation, and denature erythrocyte membranes. Feline haemoglobin is particularly susceptible to oxidative damage. **Even a single 500 mg tablet could cause toxicity in a cat.**

Risk factors

- Malnourished state.
- Anorexia.
- Concurrent treatment with enzyme-inducing drugs.

Clinical effects

Onset

Within 4 to 12 hours; liver enzymes start to rise within 24 hours.

Common signs

Signs are due to methaemoglobinaemia and include depression, weakness, vomiting, facial and paw oedema, brown mucous membranes, tachycardia, tachypnoea, dyspnoea and hypothermia.

Other signs

Haemoglobinuria, hepatic necrosis (much less common in cats) and renal damage.

Treatment

- Empty the stomach and give activated charcoal (see Decontamination).

- Acetylcysteine is an antidote that binds to toxic metabolites and acts as a glutathione precursor.
- Monitor hepatic and renal function.
- Manage methaemoglobinaemia with vitamin C, sodium sulphate (1.6% solution; 50 mg/kg bodyweight i.v. q4h, up to 24 hours) and methylthioninium chloride (methylene blue) as required.
- Oxygen for respiratory distress.
- A blood transfusion may be required for severe methaemoglobinaemia.
- Symptomatic and supportive care.

Prognosis

Guarded; treatment with acetylcysteine is effective but prompt and aggressive management is essential.

Permethrin exposure in cats

Description/Source

A pyrethroid insecticide used to prevent and treat insect infestations. Products are available for direct application on to the animal (spot-on treatments, shampoo, flea sprays, flea collars) or for treating the animal's living area (dusting powders and sprays). Exposure often occurs through accidental application of a canine spot-on preparation or through cohabitation or contact with a permethrin-treated dog or the dog's bedding.

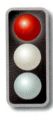

Toxicology

Permethrin alters the kinetics of voltage-dependent sodium channels in nerve membranes, which causes repetitive discharges or membrane depolarization. Cats are very susceptible, possibly due to the feline liver being relatively inefficient at glucuronide conjugation. This leads to slow excretion and the accumulation of metabolites.

Risk factors

None known.

Clinical effects

Onset

1 to 3 hours, but can be delayed for up to 36 hours.

Common signs

Vomiting, hypersalivation, ataxia, dilated pupils, tachycardia, hyperexcitability, hyperaesthesia, hyperthermia, tachypnoea, tremor, twitching, muscle fasciculations, convulsions and respiratory distress.

Other signs

Local irritation and alopecia at the site of application. Urinary retention occurs occasionally.

Treatment

- Decontaminate by washing with a mild detergent and lukewarm water (see Decontamination).
- Diazepam can be used for tremors, twitching or convulsions but other drugs will probably be required (e.g. pentobarbital, phenobarbital, propofol, methocarbamol).
- Cooling measures may be required.
- Consider use of intravenous lipid emulsion in a severe case unresponsive to other therapies.
- Symptomatic and supportive care.

Prognosis

Favourable if mild signs occur. Poor if convulsions are uncontrolled.

Petroleum distillate exposure in cats

Description/Source

Complex chemical mixtures derived from the distillation of crude oil. They include both aliphatic and aromatic hydrocarbons.

Toxicology

Irritant to skin and mucous membranes. May cause central nervous system depression if inhaled or ingested in large quantities. Severe clinical presentations result from aspiration pneumonia. The greater the volatility, the greater the risk of development of aspiration-induced pulmonary oedema.

Risk factors

None known.

Clinical effects

Onset

Usually 1 to 8 hours.

Common signs

Retching, hypersalivation, vomiting, buccal ulceration, inappetence, anorexia, abdominal tenderness and diarrhoea. Skin blisters, inflammation, burns and alopecia may occur with dermal exposure.

Other signs

Aspiration may lead to coughing, dyspnoea and pulmonary oedema. Signs can progress for the first 24–48 hours with recovery over 3–10 days. Signs of systemic poisoning include ataxia, disorientation, tremor, drowsiness and coma.

Treatment

- Gut decontamination by emesis or gastric lavage is **contraindicated** owing to aspiration risks.
- Activated charcoal is not useful.
- Decontaminate skin by washing with a mild detergent and lukewarm water (see Decontamination).
- Collar and isolate from other animals to prevent cross-contamination.
- Ensure adequate hydration.
- Symptomatic and supportive care.
- Assess respiration and check for development of pneumonitis if aspiration is suspected.

Prognosis

Favourable in most cases. Guarded if aspiration has occurred.

Piperazine exposure in cats

Description/Source

An anthelmintic used for the treatment of gastrointestinal roundworms.

Toxicology

Piperazine acts as a gamma-aminobutyric acid (GABA) agonist, causing hyperpolarization of the neuronal membrane of the worm. This results in a less excitable neuronal membrane and a decrease in nerve transmission so that the worm becomes paralysed. In mammals piperazine has effects on smooth, cardiac and skeletal muscle. Contraction of smooth muscle appears to be mediated by muscarinic cholinergic receptors. Adverse effects can occur at therapeutic doses.

Risk factors

None known.

Clinical effects

Onset

Within 12–24 hours.

Common signs
Ataxia, hypersalivation, vomiting and hyperaesthesia.

Other signs
Diarrhoea, tremor, twitching, head pressing, anorexia, dilated pupils, weakness, lethargy, hyperventilation, respiratory depression and convulsions.

Treatment
- Empty the stomach and give activated charcoal (see Decontamination).
- Symptomatic and supportive care.
- Diazepam may be used for sedation or for control of convulsions.

Prognosis
Favourable.

Praziquantel exposure in cats

For exposure in dogs – see page 86

Description/Source
Praziquantel is a prazinoisoquinoline derivative broad-spectrum anthelmintic used in the treatment of trematode and cestode infections.

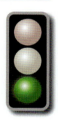

Toxicology
Praziquantel has a wide margin of safety and large doses have been tolerated in toxicity studies. The incidence of adverse effects at therapeutic doses is low. The mechanism of toxicity in mammals is unknown.

Risk factors
None known.

Clinical effects

Onset
Probably within a few hours.

Common signs
Hypersalivation, vomiting, depression and diarrhoea.

Other signs
None.

Treatment
- Gut decontamination is not required.
- Symptomatic and supportive care, if required.

Prognosis
Excellent.

Spathiphyllum species exposure in cats

Alternative names
Peace lily, white sails

Description/Source
A very popular house plant up to 1.2 metres high. The leaves are long, usually glossy or velvety, and are dark green above and paler beneath. The flowers are minute and arranged on a columnar spadix. Fruits are rarely produced by plants growing in Britain and Ireland.

Toxicology
Spathiphyllum species contain calcium oxalate crystals. Large bundles of needle-like crystals are present in specialized cells that respond to a trigger (crushing, slicing, etc.) by firing the crystals in rapid succession until the cell is empty. Although there is some controversy as to the mechanism of injury, it is generally believed that entry of the crystals into tissue facilitates the entry of other inflammatory or irritant substances.

Risk factors
None known.

Clinical effects

Onset
Variable; 1 to 24 hours.

Common signs
Hypersalivation, diarrhoea, vomiting, anorexia, lethargy, ataxia and polydipsia.

Other signs
Oral ulceration may be severe. Renal failure can occur but is rare.

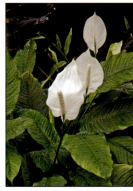

Spathiphyllum blandum.
©Elizabeth Dauncey

Treatment

- Emetics are unlikely to be required.
- Ensure adequate hydration and give anti-emetics if required.
- Check renal function in severe cases.
- Symptomatic and supportive care.

Prognosis

Favourable in most cases. Guarded in animals with renal involvement.

Toad venom exposure in cats

For exposure in dogs – see page 106

Description/Source

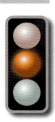

Two toads are native to Britain: the common toad (*Bufo bufo*); and the extremely rare natterjack toad (*Bufo calamita*). Most exposures occur during the summer months when toads are spawning.

Toxicology

All *Bufo* species of toads have parotid glands that secrete venom when the toad is threatened. All toads secrete similar venom; however, the toxicity of the venom varies between species. The venom contains various cardiotoxic substances, catecholamines and indole alkylamines. Serious poisonings are rare in Britain.

Risk factors

None known.

Clinical effects

Onset

Often within 30 to 60 minutes.

Common signs

Hypersalivation, frothing or foaming at the mouth, vomiting, erythematous mucous membranes, vocalizing, anxiety, ataxia and shaking.

Other signs

Twitching, tachycardia or bradycardia, hyperthermia, convulsions, coma and arrhythmias.

Treatment

- Gut decontamination is not required.

- Decontaminate the oral cavity by rinsing with water.
- Monitor pulse, respiration and temperature.
- Atropine can be used for hypersalivation or bradycardia.
- Tachycardia can be treated with beta-blockers.
- Symptomatic and supportive care.

Prognosis

Favourable.

Tramadol exposure in cats

For exposure in dogs – see page 107

Description/Source

Tramadol is an opioid analgesic used to treat mild to moderate pain.

Toxicology

Tramadol has a low affinity for opioid receptors but may have some selectivity for the mu receptor. The main analgesic effect is thought to be inhibition of the reuptake of noradrenaline and serotonin.

Risk factors

Epilepsy may increase the risk of convulsions (contraindicated in humans with epilepsy).

Clinical effects

Onset

Usually within 5 hours, but may be delayed if a sustained release preparation has been ingested.

Common signs

Frothing or foaming at the mouth, hypersalivation, drowsiness, lethargy, depression, ataxia, vomiting and dilated pupils.

Other signs

Cats may appear dysphoric or euphoric. Respiratory depression, cyanosis, hypothermia, coma and convulsions. Rarely agitation, tachycardia, tachypnoea and hyperthermia.

Treatment

- Empty the stomach and give activated charcoal (see Decontamination).

- Warming measures if required.
- Naloxone can be given for severe respiratory or central nervous system depression.
- Symptomatic and supportive care.

Prognosis

Favourable.

Yucca species exposure in cats

Description/Source

Perennial shrubs and trees, some of which are popular as houseplants. Morphology and appearance varies enormously between species. Some have spines.

Toxicology

Considered of relatively low toxicity. Some species contain saponins that may be irritant. Spines may cause mechanical injury.

Risk factors

None known.

Clinical effects

Onset

Usually within 2 to 4 hours.

Common signs

Retching, hypersalivation, diarrhoea, vomiting, inappetence and dehydration.

Other signs

Mechanical injury.

Treatment

Yucca sp.
©Elizabeth Dauncey

- Gut decontamination is not required, and *should be avoided if a spiny specimen has been ingested*.
- Ensure adequate hydration.
- Bland diet.
- Symptomatic and supportive care.

Prognosis

Excellent.

Zopiclone exposure in cats

For exposure in dogs – see page 117

Description/Source

A cyclopyrrolone hypnotic, used in the short-term treatment of insomnia in humans.

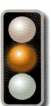

Toxicology

Zopiclone is unrelated to benzodiazepines. It acts on the neurotransmitter gamma-aminobutyric acid (GABA) receptor complex but at a different site to the benzodiazepines. It has sedative, anticonvulsant and muscle relaxant effects. The individual response is variable and not dose-related.

Risk factors

None known.

Clinical effects

Onset

Usually within 4 hours.

Common signs

Drowsiness, ataxia, lethargy and vomiting.

Other signs

Paradoxically, in some cats there may be hyperactivity, hyperaesthesia, hypersalivation, tachycardia, agitation, aggression and hyperthermia. Pupils may be dilated. Hypotension, coma and respiratory depression have been reported in human cases and could possibly occur in cats.

Treatment

- Empty the stomach and give activated charcoal (see Decontamination).
- Flumazenil could be considered in animals with severe respiratory or central nervous system depression, but is rarely required. *Dosage*: 0.01–0.02 mg/kg i.v., repeated after about 30 minutes, if required.
- Symptomatic and supportive care.

Prognosis

Favourable.

A B C D E F G H I J K L M N O P Q R S T U V W X Y Z

Case history checklist

Sadly, poisoning in animals is not an uncommon occurrence. Whilst many accidental exposures may not result in significant clinical effects or signs of intoxication, some substances pose a significant hazard to pets. Deterioration can be rapid, and speedy responses are therefore crucial. Recording as complete a case history as possible is important to ensure appropriate triage, decontamination, and efficient and optimal further management. The following is a useful checklist of information often needed to help this process for a poisoning case. There may be instances where no incident has actually been observed. In these instances this list can still be helpful.

These data, and the content of this poisons guide, should help you determine your next course of action for common potential intoxications. Treat for the worst likely possible scenario. For specific advice on decontamination procedures see pages 161–163.

Information needed	Comments
The owner	
Name and contact details	Get these at the start, in case you get cut off or lose contact. Calling back may be necessary.
The animal(s)	
Name(s)	You may have valuable past data in patient files. Ensures you are talking about the right animal(s) in multi-animal cases/households.
Species/breed	Some poisons act differently in different species and sometimes even in different breeds. Some drugs that might be used in the management of cases could be dangerous in certain species or breeds.
Age	Age or youth can affect metabolic and other physiological processes.
Sex	Sex and also whether neutered or not could affect various physiological processes. Exposures in pregnant or lactating animals may cause poisoning in the unborn or suckling offspring.
Weight	Exact if possible; best estimate if not. This enables calculation of exposure dose per kg bodyweight, which can help determine whether in toxic range, and enables doses of drugs and antidotes to be calculated correctly.

Information needed	Comments
Other medical history	Some disease states may affect responses to poisons. Current medications could interact with poison or drugs used in the treatment.
The 'poison'	
Full name	Record complete name exactly as it appears on product packaging, with ingredients if possible. Similar branding within product ranges by manufacturers can confuse. If a plant, determine common and/or Latin name (if known). Keep packaging, inserts and/or samples if available.
Manufacturer's name	In some cases this may help gather more information about the product by telephone, internet, poisons information service, etc.
Strength/ concentration of active ingredients	Vital for pharmaceutical products and pesticides.
Other composition details	Are there other formulation details, e.g. solvents, excipients? In the case of drugs, is the formulation standard or modified release?
Presentation/ packaging details	For example: bottle size, pack weights, tablets, capsules, vials, ampoules, units.
Presentation during the exposure	Concentrated/diluted? Mixed with other products? Which parts of plants/fungi?
The incident	
General	Detailed investigation of an incident can often exclude poisoning from a differential diagnosis listing. If no apparent exposure has been observed, ask the owners about medicines and products in the home and garden. Has the animal been outside? Has it been given any medicine or other treatments? Is there any evidence that plants have been eaten in the house or garden? Has it been scavenging in the dustbin, garage or shed? Does the owner live on or near agricultural land? Are any other animals in the house unwell or exposed?
Where?	Knowledge of where the incident occurred can help refine the diagnosis.

Information needed	Comments
When? Duration?	Knowing how much time has elapsed since exposure occurred may affect management options and likelihood or magnitude of exposure.
How and why?	Accidental? Suspicious/malicious? Therapeutic error? Adverse reaction?
Route(s) of exposure	For skin exposures – has the animal groomed itself and ingested poison as well?
Quantity?	Maximum/minimum values can be helpful. How much poison has been consumed or has spilt? How much, if any, is left?
The case	
Effects	What effects and/or clinical signs have occurred? Severity? How long after exposure? Are they continuing? If not, how long did they last?
Treatments/ investigations	What has been done so far by owners? By you? By others? Have samples been taken? If vomiting has occurred, is there anything in the vomit, e.g. tablets, plant material?

If the initial communication was by telephone and you later see the owner/animal, it is often useful to re-confirm details taken initially. Histories have a habit of changing!

Keep your notes! Another crucial aspect of unusual or unexpected poisonings is documentation. Where poisonings or adverse reactions relating to veterinary medicines or products occur, it is important that the necessary authorities (e.g. the UK Veterinary Medicines Directorate Suspected Adverse Reaction Surveillance Scheme, www.vmd.defra.gov.uk) and the manufacturers are notified. This should happen even if you feel the reaction or instance is known about or commonplace as such reports can lead to licences, classifications, packaging or package warnings and even manufacturing processes being reassessed or investigated.

Poisons information services like VPIS will usually follow up cases that have been referred to them, particularly where unusual or novel exposures are involved, or new management techniques have been used.

The VPIS Poisons Checklist is available as a download from the VPIS website (www.vpisglobal.com).

Decontamination

All emergency cases should initially be evaluated in the same manner with a major body systems assessment (cardiovascular, respiratory, neurological) and provided with empirical support of these systems if any is abnormal. Decontamination procedures should be initiated at the earliest possible opportunity. Key points regarding decontamination are noted below.

Dermal decontamination

- If the animal cannot undergo immediate dermal decontamination, place an Elizabethan collar to prevent grooming and oral ingestion.
- Isolate the patient from any other pets/children to prevent grooming or contamination.
- Consider carefully clipping hair, especially in long haired animals.
- Warm water and mild detergents (e.g. baby shampoo) are sufficient for most dermal contaminants.
- Contamination with oily substances may require stronger degreasing detergents such as Swarfega®. Such detergents need to be washed off thoroughly in turn.
- Take care not to induce hypothermia, especially in small patients.
- Do not use solvents such as alcohol or white spirit as this may spread the contaminant further and may irritate the skin.
- Never neutralize acids with alkalis/bases or *vice versa*.
- Ensure veterinary staff members are adequately protected by the use of plastic aprons, gloves and goggles if necessary.

Gastrointestinal decontamination

Gastrointestinal decontamination should be considered in all acute cases of toxin ingestion and generally includes gastric evacuation and administration of an adsorbent. Gastric evacuation is performed either by induction of emesis or gastric lavage. In some situations gastric evacuation is not required or recommended.

Contraindications to gastric evacuation include:

- If the ingested substance was caustic, corrosive, petroleum-based or volatile
- If the substance was ingested greater than 2 to 3 hours prior to presentation (seek advice, after this time as some substances may still be retrieved after this period).

Induction of emesis

In patients with suspected oral toxin ingestion, the induction of emesis is recommended at the earliest possible opportunity.

Contraindications to the induction of emesis include:

- If the ingested substance is caustic, acidic, volatile, petroleum or detergent based
- If the patient has severe CNS depression
- If the patient has respiratory distress
- If the poison ingested is known to cause seizures.

Remember that some emetics have a short delay before action.

Emetics cannot be used in horses, rodents, rabbits or ruminants.

There are several options for the induction of emesis:

- Apomorphine – this is the licensed product available in the UK for induction of emesis in dogs. The licensed dose is 0.1 mg/kg (s.c.). Apomorphine can however be effective when given by other routes including intramuscular, intravenous or conjunctival. The doses recommended for these routes are 0.04–0.25 mg/kg. It is a centrally acting emetic that is extremely effective in dogs but is not recommended in cats as it is variably effective.
- Xylazine (0.6 mg/kg i.m. or 1 mg/kg s.c.), dexmedetomidine (3–5 μg/kg i.m.) or medetomidine (5–20 μg/kg i.m.) – can be used in cats, although the sedative effects may be unwelcome. They are more effective if the cat's stomach is full.
- Sodium carbonate (washing soda) crystals – an effective emetic in dogs and cats. The dose is empirical but usually a large crystal in a medium- to large- breed dog and a small crystal in a small dog or cat is sufficient. Although it may be administered by the owner, caution is recommended as it is mildly caustic. It is also vital that it is not confused with caustic soda (sodium hydroxide)!
- Ropinirole (Clevor 30 mg/ml eye drops) is also licensed for induction of emesis in dogs. The dose is 2–15 μl/kg (equivalent to 1–8 drops).
- Other options such as Syrup of Ipecac, household remedies (table salt, mustard) and hydrogen peroxide are not recommended and can be dangerous.

Gastric lavage

- Gastric lavage should be performed if it is not safe to induce emesis. It is not as effective as emesis so if emesis can be safely induced this is preferred.
- Patient should be lightly anaesthetized and the trachea intubated with a cuffed endotracheal tube.
- A large bore stomach tube should be used to instil 10 ml/kg warm tap water.
- The patient's stomach should be gently agitated by manual palpation.
- The fluid should be allowed to drain by lowering the stomach tube and the patient's head.
- The procedure should be repeated (commonly 10 to 20 times) until the fluid returns relatively clear.
- This procedure will be ineffective if the material ingested is too large to pass up the tube.

Administration of adsorbents

The most commonly used adsorbent is activated charcoal. This must be administered as a powder or slurry as its effectiveness is related to its surface area.

Activated charcoal

- Activated charcoal (AC) should be administered post emesis/ gastric lavage; it acts as an adsorbent for many toxins and further reduces GI absorption.
- Slurries are more effective than tablets or capsules.
- Recommended dose is 1–4 g/kg and may be repeated every 4 to 6 hours for the first 24 to 48 hours or until charcoal is seen in the faeces.
- Repeat dose administration of AC is particularly important when the agent is enterohepatically recirculated, e.g. salicylates, barbiturates, theobromine and methylxanthines.
- AC slows GI transit time, thus co-administration of a cathartic (e.g. sorbitol or magnesium sulphate) can be considered although is not recommended in dehydrated patients or patients where there is a suspicion of ileus.
- AC use may be contraindicated if orally administered/treatments or antidotes are to be given.

Ocular decontamination

Ocular exposure is uncommon but leads to severe clinical signs, especially if there is extensive corneal damage. Alkaline damage is particularly severe and can result in deep corneal ulceration.

Ocular exposure should be managed promptly.

- As a first aid measure, owners can be advised to flush the eye with water prior to presentation at a veterinary practice, the potential severity of toxic exposure should be emphasized and the owner encouraged to attend as soon as possible.
- Contaminated eyes should be flushed with copious volumes of 0.9% saline or water for a minimum of 10 to 15 minutes.
- Sedation or anaesthesia may be required to facilitate decontamination.
- Repeated flushing may be required.
- After flushing the eye the corneal surface should be stained with fluorescein and examined carefully for ulceration.
- In the case of alkaline exposures or severe corneal damage a veterinary ophthalmologist should be contacted.
- In the case of alkaline exposure the ocular surface pH can be monitored using a urine dipstick. If the pH remains greater than 7.5 repeat flushing is recommended.
- Neutralizing agents MUST NOT be used as they may worsen damage.
- Mild corneal damage should be managed with ocular lubrication, topical antibiotics and parenteral analgesics as required.

Case submission form

You may wish to use this form to submit case details to VPIS. Contact/client/patient information is only requested to help identify the case should VPIS wish to ask for further details. All case details supplied are kept strictly confidential by VPIS. Severe or interesting cases, or those where VPIS is undertaking ongoing surveillance, referred directly to VPIS by telephone will usually be followed up by postal questionnaire as a matter of routine and so need not be submitted by this means.

YOUR NAME (REQUIRED):

YOUR EMAIL (REQUIRED):

YOUR CONTACT NUMBER:

DATE AND TIME OF PRESENTATION AT SURGERY:

ANIMAL NAME/OWNER NAME/CLIENT REFERENCE NUMBER:

ANIMAL SPECIES/BREED:

AGE:

SEX:

WEIGHT:

AGENT(S) – NAME(S) / TRADE NAME(S):

ROUTE(S) OF EXPOSURE:

AMOUNT(S):

TIME SINCE EXPOSURE:

WHEN / HOW INCIDENT OCCURRED:

LOCATION OF INCIDENT:

CLINICAL EFFECTS SEEN (including details of onset, duration, severity):

TREATMENTS INSTITUTED AND INVESTIGATIONS UNDERTAKEN:

OUTCOME (IF KNOWN):

INFORMATION AND REFERRAL SERVICES CONSULTED:

CLINICAL NOTES OR OTHER RELEVANT DOCUMENTATION ENCLOSED:	**I AM HAPPY TO BE CONTACTED BY VPIS FOR MORE DETAILS ABOUT THIS CASE:**
[ ] YES [ ] NO	[ ] YES [ ] NO

This form may be sent by post to: VPIS, 2nd Floor, Godfree Court, 29–35 Long Lane, London SE1 4PL, United Kingdom or by email to info@vpisglobal.com

Index